Management of the Patient in the Coronary Care Unit

EDITED BY

Mehdi H. Shishehbor, DO, MPH.
National Institute of Health K12 Scholar
Interventional Cardiology Fellow, Department of Cardiovascular Medicine
Cleveland Clinic
Cleveland, Ohio

Thomas H. Wang, MD
Chief Fellow, Department of Cardiovascular Medicine
Cleveland Clinic
Cleveland, Ohio

Arman T. Askari, MD
Staff, Department of Cardiovascular Medicine
Associate Director, Cardiovascular Medicine Fellowship
Cleveland Clinic
Cleveland, Ohio

Marc S. Penn, MD, PhD
Medical Director, Coronary Intensive Care Unit
Director, Bakken Heart-Brain Institute
Departments of Cardiovascular Medicine, Biomedical Engineering and Cell Biology
Cleveland Clinic
Cleveland, Ohio

Eric J. Topol, MD
Director, Scripps Translational Science Institute
Chief Academic Officer, Scripps Health
Professor of Translational Genomics
Senior Consultant, Scripps Clinic, Division of Cardiology
La Jolla, California

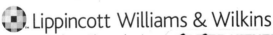 Lippincott Williams & Wilkins
a Wolters Kluwer business
Philadelphia · Baltimore · New York · London
Buenos Aires · Hong Kong · Sydney · Tokyo

Acquisitions Editor: Frances R. DeStefano
Managing Editor: Chris Potash
Developmental Editor: Jennifer Kowalak
Marketing Manager: Kim Schonberger
Project Manager: Nicole Walz
Senior Manufacturing Manager: Ben Rivera
Design Coordinator: Stephen Druding
Cover Designer: Larry Didona
Compositor: MidAtlantic Books and Journals, Inc.

Printed in the United States of America

Library of Congress Cataloging-in-Publication Data

Management of the patient in the coronary care unit / edited by Mehdi H. Shishehbor ... [et al.]. — 1st ed.
    p. ; cm.
  Includes bibliographical references and index.
  ISBN-13: 978-0-7817-6439-1 (alk. paper)
  ISBN-10: 0-7817-6439-4
  1. Cardiovascular system—Diseases—Treatment. 2. Coronary care units. 3. Health care teams. I. Shishehbor, Mehdi H.
  [DNLM: 1. Cardiovascular Diseases—diagnosis—Handbooks. 2. Cardiovascular Diseases—therapy—Handbooks. 3. Coronary Care Units—organization & administration—Handbooks. 4. Diagnosis, Differential—Handbooks. 5. Patient Care Team—organization & administration—Handbooks. WG 39 M266 2008]
  RC671.M34 2008
  362.196'1204—dc22

                        2007026684

For Susan, Sarah, and Evan
— *EJT*

For Kim, Brittany, Taylor, and Mitchell
— *MSP*

For Jamie, Alexa, Amanda, Jacob, Ali, and Houri
— *ATA*

For MiYoung, Justin, Ben, Mom and Dad.
Thanks for all your support.
— *TW*

For Andrea and Monir
— *MHS*

The fellows would also like to dedicate this book to
Eric J. Topol - for 15 years of commitment,
mentorship, and support to the fellows.
Thanks, Dr. Topol!

CONTENTS

CONTRIBUTING AUTHORS

Saif Anwaruddin, MD
Fellow, Department of
   Cardiovascular Medicine
Cleveland Clinic
Cleveland, Ohio

Alejandro C. Arroliga, MD
Director, Division of Pulmonary and
   Critical Care
Texas A&M Health Science Center
   College of Medicine
Temple, Texas

Gregory G. Bashian, MD
Electrophysiology Fellow,
   Department of Cardiovascular
   Medicine
Cleveland Clinic
Cleveland, Ohio

Mathew C. Becker, MD
Fellow, Department of
   Cardiovascular Medicine
Cleveland Clinic
Cleveland, Ohio

Sorin J. Brener, MD
Staff, Department of Cardiovascular
   Medicine
Cleveland Clinic
Cleveland, Ohio

Adnan K. Chhatriwalla, MD
Interventional Cardiology Fellow,
   Department of Cardiovascular
   Medicine
Cleveland Clinic
Cleveland, Ohio

Emily G. Chhatriwalla, RD, CNSD
Nutrition Coordinator, Intestinal
   Rehabilitation and Transplant
   Program
Cleveland Clinic
Cleveland, Ohio

Ryan D. Christofferson, MD
Interventional Cardiology Fellow,
   Department of Cardiovascular
   Medicine
Cleveland Clinic
Cleveland, Ohio

Ryan P. Daly, MD
Fellow, Department of
   Cardiovascular Medicine
Cleveland Clinic
Cleveland, Ohio

Michael G. Dickinson, MD
Staff, Heart Failure and Transplant
West Michigan Heart
Grand Rapids, Michigan

Ross A. Downey, MD
Electrophysiology Fellow,
    Department of Cardiovascular
    Medicine
Cleveland Clinic
Cleveland, Ohio

Michael D. Faulx, MD
Staff, Department of Cardiovascular
    Medicine
Cleveland Clinic
Cleveland, Ohio

Gary S. Francis, MD
Staff, Department of Cardiovascular
    Medicine
Cleveland Clinic
Cleveland, Ohio

John M. Galla, MD
Fellow, Department of
    Cardiovascular Medicine
Cleveland Clinic
Cleveland, Ohio

Adam W. Grasso, MD, PhD
Fellow, Department of
    Cardiovascular Medicine
Cleveland Clinic
Cleveland, Ohio

Brian P. Griffin, MD
Staff, Department of Cardiovascular
    Medicine
Director, Cardiovascular Medicine
    Fellowship
Cleveland Clinic
Cleveland, Ohio

Carlos A. Hubbard, MD, PhD
Fellow, Department of
    Cardiovascular Medicine
Cleveland Clinic
Cleveland, Ohio

Apur Kamdar, MD
Fellow, Department of
    Cardiovascular Medicine
Cleveland Clinic
Cleveland, Ohio

Soo H. (Esther) Kim, MD
Fellow, Department of
    Cardiovascular Medicine
Cleveland Clinic
Cleveland, Ohio

Yuli Y. Kim, MD
Fellow, Department of
    Cardiovascular Medicine
Cleveland Clinic
Cleveland, Ohio

Deborah Kwon, MD
Fellow, Department of
    Cardiovascular Medicine
Cleveland Clinic
Cleveland, Ohio

A. Michael Lincoff, MD
Staff, Department of Cardiovascular
    Medicine
Cleveland Clinic
Cleveland, Ohio

Timothy H. Mahoney, MD
Fellow, Department of
    Cardiovascular Medicine
Cleveland Clinic
Cleveland, Ohio

Telly A. Meadows, MD
Fellow, Department of
    Cardiovascular Medicine
Cleveland Clinic
Cleveland, Ohio

Venu Menon, MD
Staff, Department of Cardiovascular
  Medicine
Cleveland Clinic
Cleveland, Ohio

Michael A. Militello, PHARM.D.
Cardiology Clinical Pharmacist
Cleveland Clinic
Cleveland, Ohio

Eduardo Mireles-Cabodevila, MD
Fellow, Department of Pulmonary
  and Critical Care Medicine
Cleveland Clinic
Cleveland, Ohio

Deepu S. Nair, MD
Chief Fellow, Department of
  Cardiovascular Medicine
Cleveland Clinic
Cleveland, Ohio

Taral N. Patel, MD
Interventional Fellow, Department of
  Cardiovascular Medicine
Mid America Heart Institute—Saint
  Luke's Health System
Kansas City, Missouri

Bret A. Rogers, MD
Fellow, Department of
  Cardiovascular Medicine
Cleveland Clinic
Cleveland, Ohio

Walid Saliba, MD
Staff, Department of Cardiovascular
  Medicine
Director, Electrophysiology
  Fellowship
Cleveland Clinic
Cleveland, Ohio

Mehdi H. Shishehbor, DO,
  MPH
Interventional Cardiology Fellow,
  Department of Cardiovascular
  Medicine
Cleveland Clinic
Cleveland, Ohio

Eric J. Topol, MD
Director, Scripps Translational
  Science Institute
Chief Academic Officer, Scripps
  Health
Professor of Translational Genomics
Senior Consultant, Scripps Clinic,
  Division of Cardiology
La Jolla, California

Thomas H. Wang, MD
Chief Fellow, Department of
  Cardiovascular Medicine
Cleveland Clinic
Cleveland, Ohio

For any cardiologist or cardiologist in training, the most exciting place in a hospital is the coronary care unit. Here one sees the whole gamut of the most acutely ill patients with cardiovascular disease, including cardiogenic shock, acute aortic dissection, mechanical complications of valvular heart disease, refractory ventricular arrhythmias, pericardial tamponade, and complicated myocardial infarction. Of course, there are many other patients with conditions of lesser acuity, including those with uncomplicated acute coronary syndrome, or patients at post-intervention with high-risk coronary anatomy or compromised ventricular function. There is no doubt that the "action" is in the CCU.

In recent years, the CCU has become even more challenging, with patients, often over the age of 80 or 90, who suffer from multisystem failure, including renal, pulmonary, brain, hepatic, or resistant infection. At Cleveland Clinic, the most memorable clinical experiences I had in my 15-year tenure occurred when I was Attending in the "G20" Coronary Intensive Care Unit and working closely with the fellows. The fellows actually ran this unit, which at any point in time may have had multiple patients with intra-aortic balloon pump counterpulsation, mechanical ventilation, or intermittent dialysis. Patients were often back and forth to the cath lab or under consideration for surgery. Surely the "coronary care" unit that originated in the 1960s as a means to more efficiently deal with heart attack has been transformed into a remarkably complex, contemporary environment, and the learning that goes on there is quite extraordinary. The impact this had on the Cleveland Clinic fellows and junior faculty was so remarkable that it led them to design and author a handbook on the CCU for the medical and cardiology community.

Management of the Patient in the Coronary Care Unit contains 34 comprehensive chapters on a range of cardiac conditions and six chapters focused on interesting case presentations. Each chapter is in an outline format, with short narratives that explain the diagnostic or management decisions. There is an Acute Management box on the second page of each chapter, which provides a concise diagnosis and management algorithm for each acute cardiac condition that requires intensive care unit admission. Evidence-based strategies are incorporated with cutting-edge treatment modalities used at the Cleveland Clinic. The overall goal of each chapter is to provide an easily accessible and accurate outline for the management of emergent situations in the coronary care unit.

The first chapter provides a simple systematic approach to the CCU. This is followed by a section on acute coronary syndromes, with specific recommendations based on cutting-edge evidence, including a dedicated chapter on post-coronary intervention management. The section on acute decompensated valvular heart disease dissects each valvular condition with detailed echocardiographic and hemodynamic tips. The fourth section is on arrhythmias; it includes a number of ECG strips and tips for easy identification and appropriate management of each rhythm. The next section is on the diseases of the aorta and pericardium, including aortic dissection. The section on acute decompensated heart failure contains six chapters, including a chapter on mechanical circulatory support and cardiac transplantation and management of the acutely decompensated cardiac transplant patient. The section on procedures has step-by-step instructions and indications for various cardiac procedures. The miscellaneous section has four chapters that discuss in detail ventilator management of the cardiac patient, sedation and analgesia, nutrition, and ethics. Finally, the book ends with six unique and interesting case presentations, with diagnostic and management tips.

The fellows of the "G20" CCU who have put together this manual and teaching guide deserve special recognition for their herculean efforts. Their only real incentive to do this work was to help future trainees in cardiology, medical residents, medical students, and the para-professional medical community. It is hoped that their pragmatic approach in relating what they learned to help the next generation of CCU care providers and ultimately patients will have a lasting impact as a learning and educational guide. For me, working with the fellows will always remain the most important, enjoyable, and exhilarating experience of my career.

Eric J. Topol, MD

Director, Scripps Translational Science Institute
Chief Academic Officer, Scripps Health
Professor of Translational Genomics, TSRI

Approach to Cardiac Care Unit Patient

CHAPTER 1

Approach to the Cardiac Care Unit (CCU) Patient

MEHDI H. SHISHEHBOR

THOMAS H. WANG

INTRODUCTION

Patients admitted to the cardiac care unit (CCU) are typically very sick and require immediate attention. We recommend a team-based approach. In general, we obtain as much history as possible before the patient arrives. Similarly, prior to arrival all necessary equipment should be ready (i.e., A-line, echo machine, etc). We have outlined the pertinent information that should be obtained prior to the patient's arrival, upon examination in the CCU, and during his or her stay. Additionally, we have provided useful templates to be carried on rounds.

Preadmission

Obtain as much history as possible from the referring physician. For example, a history of ascending aortic dissection would require that the surgical team be notified prior to patient arrival. Appropriate medications such as sodium nitroprusside and labetalol should be ready, and an ECG, echo, and CXR should be on standby for patient arrival. Clear communication between the referring physician and the CCU personnel can save time and lives.

The following are important factors when accepting a patient to the CCU:

1. Name and the number of the referring physician
2. Primary diagnosis
3. Level of consciousness
4. Vitals (blood pressure, heart rate, respiratory rate, and oxygenation)

5. Current medications
6. Most recent labs (specifically, serum creatinine, hemoglobin, hematocrit, platelet, INR, PT, PTT)
7. Specific labs relevant to primary diagnosis (i.e., cardiac enzymes for a patient with ACS)
8. Allergies
9. X-ray films, catheterization and echocardiography films, and reports
10. Power of attorney and do-not-resuscitate (DNR) status

Admission to the CCU

Once the patient arrives, a team-based approach is ideal. In our CCU, the nursing team, respiratory therapist, residents, and fellows work together to stabilize the patient. We recommend the following approach:

1. One individual should obtain data from the chart and old records.
2. The nursing team should obtain at least two large IVs and blood should be drawn and sent for routine labs.
3. An ECG, CXR should be immediately performed.
4. While the other members of the team are performing these tasks, the senior physician should examine the patient, obtain a quick history, and take appropriate measures to stabilize the patient.
5. Once a preliminary assessment is performed, decisions regarding consultations and other procedures should be made.
6. After the initial work up, the resident/medical student responsible for the care of the patient should examine the patient very carefully. Any heart murmur or abnormality should be documented.
7. An echocardiogram should be routinely performed immediately. This is typically done by the cardiology fellow.
8. Invasive procedures such as right-heart catheterization, IABP, temporary pacemakers, and even Quinton catheters should be performed under fluoroscopy in a designated procedure room, if possible.
9. For all admissions to the CCU, a full cardiac history including the coronary anatomy, presence of valvular disease, left-ventricular function, and prior open-heart surgeries should be obtained.

During the CCU Stay

We have provided two templates, based on our work at the Cleveland Clinic, to aid in the daily management of the medications, labs, and procedural results for each patient (Table 1.1). Careful attention must be

Table 1.1   Admission to the CCU

Name

Clinic #

Allergies

Date of Admit

Date of Admit to CCU

PMHx

HPI

Cardiac Cath

Echo

PSHx

Nuclear/CT/MRI

Social Hx

Date																			
ASA																			
Plavix																			
Statin																			
Beta-bl																			
ACE-I																			
GI ppx																			
DVT ppx																			

Table 1.1 Admission to the CCU (continued)

Date	Date	Date	Date	Date	Date	Date
Time						
CK						
MB						
MB%						
Trop						

Table 1.1   Admission to the CCU (continued)

	Date	Date	Date
Na			
K			
Cl			
HCO3			
BUN	Date	Date	Date
Cr			
Gluc			
WBC			
Hbg			
HCT			
Plt	Date	Date	Date
INR			
Ptt			
Mg			
Ca			
Phos			
TP			

Table 1.1 Admission to the CCU (continued)

	Date	Date	Date
Alb			
T bili			
AST			
ALT			
Alk ph			
	Date	Date	Date
	Date	Date	Date

Table 1.1	Admission to the CCU (continued)									
Date	Date	Date	Date	Date	Date	Date	Date	Date	Date	
Bld cx										
Ur cx										
Sput cx										
Line cx										

paid to these details to ensure optimal patient management. We recommend that each patient's echocardiogram result and coronary anatomy be known at all times and signed out to covering physicians.

Rounding on Patients

In addition to daily rounds with the staff, the CCU team should routinely round continuously as time permits. We recommend a systematic approach as outlined here:

1. Briefly review the patient's history and physical. This is very helpful in guiding your thought process as you review the data and the medications. Furthermore, this will help with titrating medications.

2. Start with the nurse's flow sheet— review the hemodynamic data and remember to focus on trends as opposed to an isolated number. The next step is to note the intake and output over the last 24 hours and during the hospitalization. This is extremely important in cardiac patients, especially in postcardiac catheterization and heart-failure patients. Subsequently, review all intravenous (IV) and by mouth (PO) medications.

3. Check labs.

4. Utilize a systems-based approach when developing a plan for the patient. For cardiovascular issues, be sure to address blood pressure, lipid profile, anticoagulation, rhythm issues, imaging tests, and risk stratification. Also, be certain to address GI prophylaxis, DVT prophylaxis, nutrition, and skin care (i.e., decubitus ulcers).

5. Check dates on IVs and central lines.

6. Depending on each patient's history and physical, develop a task list based on the plan developed.

Things to Know on Rounds

1. Events within the last 24 hours including total intake and output, hemodynamic trends, and therapeutic interventions such as medications or procedures

2. Cardiac risk factors

3. Lab values such as cardiac enzymes, lipid levels, HgbA1C, BMP, CBC, PT, INR, PTT, and any other tests that were ordered

4. Left ventricular and valvular function as well as coronary anatomy (i.e., any prior PCI or CABG, location, type, and length of stents)

5. Date IVs and lines were placed

6. A systems-based plan of action

Acute Coronary Syndromes

CHAPTER 2

Acute ST-Elevation Myocardial Infarction

RYAN D. CHRISTOFFERSON

ST-elevation myocardial infarction (STEMI) is a true medical emergency. On a spectrum of acute ischemic syndromes, STEMI is thought to represent transmyocardial injury from complete occlusion of an epicardial coronary artery. The first step to proper management of STEMI is prompt recognition of the problem, which requires a critical assessment of the clinical presentation and ECG.

Initial efforts should be directed toward timely reperfusion of the infarct-related artery, either by primary percutaneous coronary intervention (PCI) or fibrinolytics, with primary PCI as the preferred treatment when available. The central paradigm in the management of STEMI is "time is myocardium." After a reperfusion strategy has been chosen and executed, the subsequent course in the coronary care unit (CCU) will largely depend on whether or not the infarct-related artery was opened in a timely fashion and the presence or absence of left-ventricular (LV) dysfunction. For patients with early and complete reperfusion, the CCU stay is often short (generally 1 night) and uncomplicated. However, for patients with incomplete, late or no reperfusion, or severe left- or right-ventricular dysfunction, the CCU stay may be long and arduous. During this phase of management, the focus becomes the application of proper medical therapy (Chapter 6) and surveillance for complications of myocardial infarction (Chapter 4).

ACUTE MANAGEMENT

Diagnostic Tests:

- **ECG:** 12-lead at presentation, repeat after initial medical therapy
- **CXR:** Portable to assess cardiac and aortic silhouette for aneurysm/dissection
- **TTE:** To assess for wall motion abnormalities, in particular if diagnosis uncertain, and identify complications of MI such as mitral regurgitation or papillary muscle rupture. (This should not delay transfer to cardiac catheterization laboratory or fibrinolytic therapy.)

Management:

Initial Labs: CBC, CMP, PT, PTT, Troponin, CK, CK-MB, type, and screen

Medications:

- **On Presentation:**
  - Aspirin 325 mg PO immediately
  - Oxygen to keep sat ≥90%
  - Atorvastatin 80 mg/daily
  - Nitroglycerin 0.4 mg SL immediately, followed by nitroglycerin gtt @10 to 20 µg/min and titrate if blood pressure above 100mmHg (Use with caution in patients with inferior infarction and avoid in those with right ventricular infarction).
  - IV (intravenous) unfractionated heparin 60 units/kg bolus followed by 12 units/kg infusion.
  - Consider metoprolol 5 mg IV q5 minutes until desired heart rate is reached (Avoid in patients with Killip class II, III, IV)– Clopidogrel 300 to 600 mg orally.

Tools:

- Pulmonary artery catheter: useful for cardiogenic shock or hemodynamic instability
- Intra-aortic balloon pump: for refractory chest pain, arrhythmia, or hemodynamic compromise

Primary Percutaneous Coronary Intervention (PCI) versus Fibrinolytics

Primary PCI favored if available immediately or transfer time to referral center is timely (<3 hours), if late presentation (>3 hours chest pain), or if severe heart failure or contraindication to fibrinolytics are present
* Load clopidogrel 600 mg by mouth (PO) on the way to catheterization laboratory
* Order weight-based abciximab bolus (0.25 mg/kg) and drip (0.125 µg/kg/min)

Thrombolytics favored if early presentation (<3 hours chest pain) and primary PCI is unavailable or prolonged transfer time anticipated (>3 hours)
* t-PA (if weight >67 kg total dose = 15 mg IV bolus then 50 mg over 30 minutes then 35 mg over 60 minutes), streptokinase (1.5 million IU over 60 minutes) or
* Tenecteplase (single IV bolus over 5 seconds)—see dosing below
* Reteplase 10 units over 2 minutes then 10 units again after 30 minutes
* Heparin 40 to 50 units/kg bolus and followed by 12 units/kg gtt

CCU Tip

Initiate smoking cessation counseling, intensive lipid-lowering therapy, beta blocker, and angiotensin converting enzyme inhibitor while patient still in cardiac intensive care unit (CICU). Any hemodynamic instability could potentially be a complication of MI.

PRESENTATION

Patients who present with STEMI typically have a prior history of angina or coronary artery disease, are elderly, and are most frequently males. Events typically cluster in the morning hours, coincident with activation of the neurohormonal and sympathetic nervous system. The clinical presentation of STEMI does vary, but typically the history begins with the sudden onset of severe precordial chest pain or dyspnea. Patients typically describe a crushing, squeezing, or pressure sensation, often in a retrosternal location, with or without radiation to the neck, jaw, left shoulder, or left arm. Physicians should be aware that many patients, however, present with atypical symptoms, including arm or shoulder pain, acute dyspnea only, syncope, or arrhythmias. It is unusual for patients to present with STEMI in the absence of symptoms, a finding that should raise suspicion for other causes of ST elevation besides myocardial injury.

PHYSICAL EXAMINATION

An important aspect of the physical examination is a careful assessment for signs or symptoms of impending cardiac failure. The Killip classification may be useful for evaluating the hemodynamic significance of the myocardial injury and can confer important prognostic information (Table 2.1).

- General: anxious, distressed, diaphoretic, Levine's sign (clenched fist on chest), often normotensive or hypertensive
- Neck: normal or mildly elevated jugular venous pressure (JVP)
- Cardiac: tachycardia, soft S1, S4 present, possible S3 present, systolic murmur
- Lungs: potentially rales and wheezing if LV failure present
- Extremities: normal or signs of peripheral vascular disease

DIFFERENTIAL DIAGNOSIS

There are three major types of differential diagnostic considerations for STEMI (Table 2.2). First, there are a number of problems that can produce STEMI as a comorbid condition, an example being acute aortic dissection where the dissection flap extends into the left main coronary

Table 2.1	Killip classification in the GUSTO-1 trial.	
Killip Class	Clinical Characteristics	30-day Mortality (%)
I	No evidence of CHF	5.1
II	Rales, jugular venous distention or S3	13.6
III	Pulmonary edema	32.2
IV	Cardiogenic shock	57.8

CHF, chronic heart failure

Table 2.2	Differential diagnostic considerations for ST-elevation myocardial infarction.		
Conditions with comorbid coronary ischemia	**Conditions with ST elevation but no ischemia**	**Conditions with chest pain but no ischemia**	
Acute aortic dissection	Early repolarization	Acute aortic dissection	
Systemic arterial embolism: — atrial fibrillation — endocarditis — patent foramen ovale	Left ventricular hypertrophy	Myopericarditis	
Hypertensive crisis	LBBB	Pleuritis	
Aortic stenosis	Hyperkalemia	Pulmonary embolism	
Cocaine use	Brugada syndrome	Costochondritis	
Arteritis		Gastrointestinal disorders — reflux esophagitis — esophageal spasm — gastritis — cholecystitis	

artery or, more commonly, the right coronary artery. The second grouping contains conditions that present with a suspicious ECG but are not STEMI, such as acute pericarditis, where diffuse ST elevations and PR depression mimic STEMI.

Finally, there are conditions that produce chest pain in the absence of myocardial ischemia, such as pulmonary embolism. The history remains crucial for accurate diagnosis.

RISK FACTORS

- Hypertension
- Hyperlipidemia
- Tobacco use
- Dyslipidemia
- Genetic susceptibility

- Vascular inflammation
- Thrombolysis in myocardial infarction (TIMI) risk score for STEMI:

Variables	Points	Risk Score	30 day Mortality
Age ≥75	3	0	0.8
Age 65–74	2	1	1.6
Diabetes, hypertension, or angina	1	2	2.2
Systolic blood pressure <100 mmHg	3	3	4.4
Heart rate >100 beats per minute	2	4	7.3
Killip Class II–IV	2	5	12
Weight <67 kg (150 lb)	1	6	16
Anterior STEMI or complete left bundle branch block (CLBBB)	1	7	23
Time to treatment >4 hours	1	8	27

DIAGNOSTIC TESTS

The majority of diagnoses of acute ST-segment elevation myocardial infarction, as previously discussed, are made on the basis of a suspicious clinical syndrome with a diagnostic ECG. Additional diagnostic tests are utilized to diagnose or prevent complications, to aid in establishing prognosis, or to exclude comorbid conditions leading to myocardial infarction (MI).

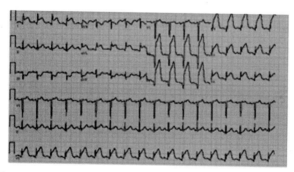

FIGURE 2.1. Anterior lateral STEMI with reciprocal changes.

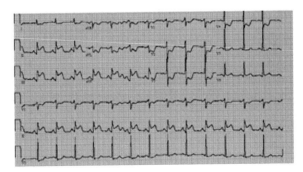

FIGURE 2.2. Inferior posterior STEMI.

ECG is necessary for the recognition of STEMI, although a new left-bundle branch block (LBBB) in the same clinical setting is a diagnostic equivalent. ST elevation refers to the number of millimeters greater voltage in the ST segment relative to the TP segment. A diagnostic ECG is generally considered to be one with 1-mm ST-segment elevation in two or more consecutive limb leads (I, II, III, AVF, AVL, AVR or 2-mm elevation in two or more consecutive precordial leads (V1–V6). It is normal to have some degree of ST elevation (1 to 2 mm) in one or more precordial leads, a finding that is most common in young men and decreases with age. Often termed "early repolarization," this finding is usually associated with most marked ST elevation in V4, a notch at the J point (the junction between the QRS complex and the ST segment), and a "concave-up" ST segment. The deeper the S wave, the greater the ST-segment elevation in this normal variant, similar to LV hypertrophy.

Transthoracic echocardiography (TTE) can be used early after presentation if the ECG is indeterminate or the diagnosis is uncertain. Lack of regional wall-motion abnormalities can potentially exclude the diagnosis. The TTE is also useful to determine LV function, which may influence prognosis and subsequent treatment options. Valvular abnormalities are common, with aortic stenosis and mitral regurgitation being most important. If not performed early in the presentation, a subsequent ECG can be useful to determine infarct size or detect complications of myocardial infarction, such as ventricular-free wall rupture or ventricular septal defect (Chapter 4).

Myocardial perfusion imaging is not useful in the acute setting; however, it may be employed subsequently to assess infarct size and residual ischemia after reperfusion.

Cardiac biomarkers are useful to aid in diagnosis, assessment of infarct size, and for prognostication. There are two biomarkers of particular utility: troponin and creatine kinase myocardial band (CK-MB). Troponin I or T is elevated early in myocardial infarction and is more useful for diagnosis, but its utility in quantifying infarct size remains under investigation. The CK-MB is useful both for diagnosis and for assessment of infarct size.

Cardiac catheterization is performed as part of an invasive reperfusion strategy (primary PCI) and can determine the infarct-related artery, as well as detail the remaining coronary anatomy. Even in patients with a pharmacologic reperfusion strategy, angiography with coronary intervention may be performed immediately after administration of fibrinolytics (facilitated PCI) or early after the event in the case of inadequate ST-segment reperfusion (rescue PCI). Facilitated PCI has been associated with increased bleeding. If ischemia is documented clinically (recurrent chest pain or ST-segment changes) or by low-level exercise or pharmacologic stress test, then acute angiography is mandated prior to discharge.

MEDICAL/INTERVENTIONAL MANAGEMENT

The initial therapeutic goal is timely reperfusion. The primary decision to be made is between fibrinolytic therapy versus primary PCI. Primary PCI is favored if this therapy is available immediately or transfer to a referral center can be accomplished in a timely fashion (<3 hours). In addition, PCI is favored if there is a late presentation (>3 hours chest pain) or if severe heart failure or contraindication to fibrinolytics are present. Fibrinolytics are favored when the patient presents early (<3 hours chest pain) and primary angioplasty is unavailable or if a prolonged transfer time is anticipated (>3 hours).

Primary Angioplasty
• Load clopidogrel 600 mg PO on way to catheterization laboratory.
• Heparin bolus 70 to 100 U/kg.
• Order weight-based abciximab abciximab bolus (0.25 mg/kg) and drip (0.125 µg/kg/min) to be sent to catheterization laboratory.

Fibrinolytic Therapy
• t-PA, reteplase, streptokinase, or tenecteplase

Lytic agent	Dose
Alteplase (tpa)	— Patient >67 kg total dose = 100 mg, 15 mg IV bolus then 50 mg over 30 minutes then 35 mg over 60 minutes.
	— Patient ≤67 kg total dose <100 mg, 15 mg IV bolus then 0.75 mg/kg over 30 minutes then 0.5 mg/kg over 60 minutes
Reteplase (rPA)	— 10 units over 2 minutes followed by a second 10-unit bolus in 30 minutes
Streptokinase (SK)	— 1.5 million IU over 60 minutes
Tenecteplase (TNK-ase)	— Single IV bolus given over 5 seconds

Weight	Dose (mg)
<60	30
≥60–<70	35
≥70–<80	40
≥80–<90	45
≥90	50

- Heparin bolus and drip
- Clopidogrel 600 mg loading dose

Postreperfusion Medical Therapy

Aspirin 81 mg/day should be taken for life.

Clopidogrel (Plavix) 600 mg loading dose should be taken followed by 75 mg/day. In our institution, all patients who receive drug-eluting stents continue with clopidogrel for at least 2 years. Those who receive bare-metal stents continue with clopidogrel for at least 1 year.

Beta blockers should be initiated in all patients without contraindications who present with STEMI within the first 24 hours and in most cases should be continued for life. We start with short-acting agents such as lopressor; once the optimum dose has been reached depending on the desired heart rate and blood pressure, a once-a-day long-acting agent such as Toprol XL should be considered. In patients with LV dysfunction, we prefer carvedilol 3.25 mg twice daily to be titrated as tolerated. Beta blockers should be avoided in patients presenting with

STEMI who are in Killip class II, III, or IV or in those with hypotension, bradycardia, or shock.

Angiotensin converting enzyme (ACE) inhibitors should also be initiated within the first 24 hours. Again, we prefer short-acting agents (captopril) in the first 24 hours until the appropriate maximum dose has been reached. Once a patient can tolerate this dose, we convert to a comparable long-acting agent such as lisinopril. ACE inhibitors should be continued for life in patients with ejection fractions less than 40% and for at least 1 month in all patients. Initiation of ACE inhibitors has been associated with early rise in creatinine; however, in most cases this is a transient phenomenon. In patients with contraindication to ACE inhibitors angiotensin receptor blockers should be considered.

Insulin therapy is recommended for tight glucose control for all patients in the cardiac intensive care unit (CICU). Data from DIGAMI and other studies support intensive glucose control in these patients. We recommend an insulin-drip algorithm for patients with two blood-glucose levels greater than 200 mg/dL. Avoid glucophage pre- and post-PCI, as this agent has been associated with lactic acidosis in this setting.

Statins should be initiated after reperfusion once the patient is hemodynamically stable. Based on the recent high-dose statin trials, we initially start most patients on atorvastatin 80 mg/day. Low-density lipoprotein cholesterol (LDL-C) should be reduced to 60 to 70 mg/dL in all patients presenting with STEMI. However, there is some evidence that high-dose statin therapy has pleiotropic effects that go beyond LDL-C level.

Amiodarone can be considered in patients with dysrrhythmias. We make every effort to avoid amiodarone in young patients. In general, aggressive beta-blocker therapy is adequate for post-MI arrhythmias.

SURGICAL MANAGEMENT

It is uncommon to undertake immediate surgical management for STEMI when the presentation is uncomplicated due to the need for early and immediate revascularization.

However, after early efforts at catheter-based or fibrinolytic-induced reperfusion are undertaken, persistent or recurrent chest pain, high-risk coronary anatomy (e.g., left-main stenosis or triple-vessel disease in a diabetic) or mechanical complication of MI (e.g., ventricular-septal defect, papillary muscle rupture) may lead to surgical consultation. In this setting, it may be more favorable to wait at least 24 hours after STEMI and after the patient is hemodynamically stable. Mechanical support from intra-aortic balloon pump may be necessary as a bridge to surgery in cases of refractory chest pain, arrhythmia, or hemodynamic instability.

COMPLICATIONS

The most common complications of myocardial infarction and their management are detailed in Chapter 4.

- Tachyarrhythmia
- Ventricular tachycardia
- Ventricular fibrillation
- Accelerated idioventricular rhythm
- Atrial fibrillation/flutter
- Bradyarrhythmia
- Junctional escape rhythm
- Atrioventricular block
- Free wall rupture
- Ventricular septal defect
- Mitral regurgitation
- Ischemic tethering of the papillary muscle
- Papillary muscle rupture
- Cardiogenic shock
- Right ventricular myocardial infarction

DISCHARGE

The patient should remain in the intensive care unit (ICU) for 12 to 24 hours after primary PCI or fibrinolytic therapy in the case of complete reperfusion to assess for complications of MI or reperfusion arrhythmia. If there is inadequate reperfusion or no reperfusion, or in the case of significant myocardial dysfunction and/or cardiogenic shock, a prolonged ICU stay may be necessary. Oral medications for blood pressure and heart-rate control, determinants of myocardial-oxygen demand, should be initiated while in the ICU, and continued on discharge to the regular nursing floor. Patients with ongoing ischemia, particularly those with recurrent chest pain, should not be transferred to the regular nursing floor prior to resolution of this issue.

RECOMMENDED READING

1. Antman EM, Braunwald E. ST-elevation myocardial infarction: pathology, pathophysiology, and clinical features. In: DP Zipes, E Braunwald, eds. *Braunwald's Heart Disease: A Textbook of Cardiovascular Medicine.* Philadelphia: WB Saunders; 2005:1141–1165.
2. Antman EM. ST-elevation myocardial infarction: management. In: DP Zipes, E. Braumwald, eds. *Braunwald's Heart Disease: A Textbook of Cardiovascular Medicine.* Philadelphia: WB Saunders; 2005:1167–1226.
3. Vivekananthan DP, Lauer MA. Acute myocardial infarction. In: Griffin, BP, Topol, EJ, eds. *Manual of Cardiovascular Medicine.* Philadelphia: Lippincott Williams & Wilkins; 2004:3–26.
4. Antman EM, Anbe DT, Armstrong PW, et al. ACC/AHA guidelines for the management of patients with ST-elevation myocardial infarction; a report of the American College of Cardiology/American Heart Association Task Force on practice guidelines (committee to revise the 1999 Guidelines for the management of patients with acute myocardial infarction). *J Am Col Cardiol.* 2004; 44:E1–E211.
5. Topol EJ. *Textbook of Cardiovascular Medicine.* 3rd ed. Lippincott Williams & Wilkins; 2007.

CHAPTER **3**

Non-ST-Segment Elevation Myocardial Infarction

CARLOS A. HUBBARD

Non-ST-segment elevation myocardial infarction (NSTEMI) is part of a wider definition of the acute coronary syndrome (ACS). NSTEMI involves nontransmural myocardial infarction with myocyte necrosis without ECG findings of ST-segment elevation myocardial infarction (MI), posterior MI, or new left bundle branch block (LBBB). NSTEMI is difficult to distinguish from unstable angina as clinical presentation, physical exam and ECG findings are not diagnostic of NSTEMI. NSTEMI is primarily diagnosed by the presence of elevated serum cardiac biomarkers.

PRESENTATION

Patients can present with typical symptoms of unstable angina (chest pain at rest or with minimal exertion, new onset, or accelerating chest pain) or atypical symptoms (nausea/vomiting, diaphoresis, back or abdominal pain), which can be more common in women, the elderly, and diabetics. Congestive heart failure (CHF) and cardiac arrhythmias are also common presentations in patients with NSTEMI.

PHYSICAL EXAM

- Heart failure
- Elevated jugular venous pressure (JVP)
- S_3 or S_4 gallop
- Pulmonary edema (rales)
- Peripheral edema

ACUTE MANAGEMENT

Diagnostic Tests:

- **ECG:** Evaluate for ST changes, deep symmetrical precordial T-wave inversions, arterioventricular block, arrhythmias; repeat serially and especially with changes in chest pain.
- **TTE:** Evaluate left- and right-ventricular function, wall motion abnormalities, pericardial effusions, septal defects, aortic root dissection, and valvular regurgitation (especially mitral insufficiency).
- **CXR:** evaluate for cardiomegaly and signs of congestive failure such as pulmonary edema, Kerley B lines, cephalization, etc.

Management:

- **Tools:** Two large-bore IV lines
- **STAT labs:** CBC, CMP, PT, PTT, TSH, BNP, CRP on admission; CK, MB, Troponin every 8 hours × 24 hours; fasting lipid panel next morning

Medications:

- Aspirin: Four chewable 81 mg tablets immediately; then 81 mg daily
- Clopidogrel: 600 mg immediately then 75 mg daily (if prompt surgical intervention unlikely in next 5 to 7 days)
- Heparin: unfractionated heparin 60 u/kg bolus (max 5,000 u) and 12 u/kg/hour (adjust per aPTT every 6 hours).
- Beta blocker: metoprolol tartrate 5 mg IV every 5 minutes until SBP <110 and HR <70; then start 25 mg by mouth every 12 hours (titrate to above goals); avoid if signs of heart failure present
- IV Nitroglycerin: start at 10 µg/min (titrate up until SBP <110 and chest pain free)
- Statin: atorvastatin 80 mg daily
- ACE inhibitor: if no renal dysfunction and blood pressure is adequate start with low-dose captopril 6.25 mg three times a day and titrate as tolerated
- Glycoprotein IIb/IIIa inhibitor: start eptifibatide 180 µg/kg bolus followed by 2 µg/kg/min infusion (renal dosing 180 µg/kg bolus; 1 µg/kg/min infusion) if the patient is high risk
- consider abciximab 0.25 mg/kg bolus and 0.125 µg/kg/min (max 10 µg/kg/min) infusion if patient is proceeding immediately to

coronary angiography andintervention (abciximab is contraindicated for medical management of ACS).
- IABP: utilize in patients with unremitting pain or dynamic ST changes despite maximal medical therapy

ACS patients with renal insufficiency:
- N-acetylcysteine: 600 mg by mouth every 12 hours 1 day prior and 2 to 3 days after
- Sodium bicarbonate infusion: (150 meq in 1 L D5W) at 3.2 mL/kg/hr for 1 hour precath and 1.8 mL/kg/hr for 6 hours postcath

Recommended consults:
- Cardiac rehabilitation
- Nutrition counseling
- Smoking cessation if indicated

CCU Tip: Opiates may mask ongoing ischemic pain and delay initiation of early invasive strategy when indicated. Select short-acting medications as hemodynamic compromise can occur suddenly. Beta blockers should be initiated carefully in the setting of heart failure, conduction abnormalities, or respiratory disease.

DIFFERENTIAL DIAGNOSIS

Cardiac
- Pericarditis
- Myocarditis

Noncardiac
- Costochondritis
- Pneumonia
- Pneumothorax
- Pulmonary embolus
- Aortic dissection
- Esophageal spasm
- Cholecystitis

Secondary Myocardial Ischemia without Critical Coronary Artery Stenosis
- Anemia
- Sepsis

Table 3.1	Risk scores.
Risk Score	14-day Death/MI/Urgent Revasc
0/1	5
2	8
3	13
4	20
5	26
6/7	41

MI, myocardial infarction

- Hypovolemia
- Hypertensive crisis
- Thyrotoxicosis

RISK FACTORS

New onset or accelerated angina convey particular risk for significant CAD. The TIMI 7-variable risk score is a validated model for risk stratification of patients with UA/NSTEMI. The presence of each variable confers cumulative risk of death, nonfatal MI or revascularization at 14 days after presentation and helps to differentiate low-, medium- and high-risk patients (Tables 3.1 and 3.2).

Table 3.2	TIMI risk score variables.
Variables	Points
Age ≥65	1
≥3 CAD risk factors	1
Known CAD (stenosis ≥50%)	1
ASA use in past 7 days	1
Recent (≤24 hours) severe angina	1
Cardiac markers positive	1
ST deviation ≥0.5 mm	1

CAD, coronary artery disease; ASA, aspirin

DIAGNOSTIC TESTS

ECG findings can be suggestive but nonspecific, and many patients with NSTEMI have no appreciable ECG changes (~20%). Signs to look for include ST-segment deviation (elevation or depression) ≥0.5 mm, development of a LBBB, or deep (≥2 mm) and symmetrical precordial T-wave inversions.

CXR should be obtained to look for signs of heart failure such as Kerley B lines, cephalization, or pulmonary edema.

Cardiac biomarkers such as creatine kinase (CK), the MB isoenzyme of CK (CK-MB), troponin I and troponin T are myocyte-specific proteins. Serum elevations of these proteins correlate well with risk of death and MI, but they can be elevated by conditions other than ACS (see Differential Diagnosis p. 29, this chapter). They should be measured serially every 8 hours for 24 hours as the markers differ in time to peak level and time to clearance after reperfusion (Table 3.3).

Echocardiography may identify specific wall-motion abnormalities associated with acute ischemia/infarction, but its sensitivity is greatly diminished by preexisting ventricular dysfunction or wall-motion abnormalities. However, it can be extremely useful in diagnosing ischemic valvular regurgitation or in evaluating intracardiac shunts.

MEDICAL MANAGEMENT

The central goals of NSTEMI treatment are to inhibit platelet activation and aggregation, inhibit thrombus formation, and provide antianginal therapy.

Antiplatelets

Aspirin should be given immediately upon presentation unless contraindicated (active bleeding, documented hypersensitivity reaction) and

Table 3.3	Cardiac biomarkers.

Cardiac biomarker	Time to peak level	Duration of elevation
Creatine kinase (CK)	12–24 h	2–3 d
CK-MB isoenzyme	10–18 h	2–3 d
Troponin T	18–24 h	10–14 d
Troponin I	18–24 h	10–14 d

MI, myocardial infarction

acts as an inhibitor of platelet aggregation by irreversible binding of cyclooxygenase in the thromboxane A2 pathway. The recommended initial dose is 325 mg chewable followed by 81 mg daily. It has a rapid onset of action (<60 minutes) and durable effect (7 to 10 days).

Clopidogrel inhibits adenosine diphosphate-mediated platelet aggregation; the major adverse effect is increased major bleeding after coronary artery bypass graft (CABG). Thus, clopidogrel should be stopped 5 to 7 days before CABG. Clopidogrel is preferable to ticlopidine due to its faster onset of action, less-frequent dosing, and better side-effect profile (ticlopidine is associated with neutropenia and TTP). The loading dose for which there is the most evidence is 300 mg, although many physicians use 600 mg to achieve more rapid platelet inhibition.

Platelet glycoprotein IIb/IIIa inhibitors inhibit platelet aggregation by blocking the surface glycoprotein IIb/IIIa receptors, which bind to fibrinogen and allow for platelet cross-linking and activation. These agents have been primarily shown to benefit patients undergoing percutaneous coronary intervention (PCI), diabetics, and patients with elevated cardiac troponins. The data for the use of these drugs were established in trials that did not use clopidogrel, so it is unclear whether IIb/IIIa inhibitors given IV provide incremental efficacy with clopidogrel in the treatment of ACS.

Abciximab (Reopro) is recommended only for patients who are undergoing PCI, and is not recommended for patients undergoing conservative therapy. It is usually initiated when the patient is in the cath lab (bolus 0.25 mg/kg IV; maintenance 10 μg/min IV—12 hours max).

Tirofiban (Aggrastat) is recommended for patients with UA/ NSTEMI in addition to aspirin and heparin regardless of whether or not they proceed to PCI (bolus 0.6 μg/kg/min IV for 30 minutes; maintenance 0.15 μg/kg/min for 24 to 36 hours—renal clearance use $1/2$ dose for CrCl <30 cc/min).

Eptifibatide (Integrilin) is recommended for patients with UA/ NSTEMI in addition to aspirin and heparin regardless of whether or not they proceed to PCI (bolus 180 μg/kg; maintenance 2.0 μg/kg/min for 72 to 96 hours). Dose adjustment should be utilized for decreased creatinine clearance.

Antianginals

Beta blockers reduce cardiac workload and oxygen consumption by decreasing heart rate and myocardial contractility and blunting the adrenergic response. Initiate metoprolol 5 mg intravenously every 5 minutes as needed to reach goal systolic blood pressure of <110 and/or heart rate of <70. Concurrently, begin metoprolol tartrate 25 to 50 mg by mouth every 6 hours for greater duration of effect.

Nitrates reduce cardiac preload, ventricular wall stress, and therefore myocardial oxygen demand. Their use is indicated for anginal symptoms, and they are also useful in the treatment of dyspnea related to pulmonary edema. Initiate therapy with sublingual nitroglycerin 0.4 mg every 5 minutes times three doses and 1 inch of topical nitroglycerin paste if anginal symptoms have resolved. If anginal symptoms persist, intravenous nitroglycerin should be initiated at 10 to 20 µg/min and titrated based on symptoms and blood pressure.

Narcotics have not been shown to favorably affect morbidity/mortality associated with UA/NSTEMI. Additionally, narcotics may mask symptoms indicative of ongoing ischemia and delay initiation of therapy.

Supplemental oxygen increases myocardial oxygen supply but without a demonstrated reduction in morbidity/mortality associated with UA/NSTEMI. It is recommended for respiratory distress and hypoxia by ACC/AHA guidelines.

Antithrombotics

Unfractionated heparin (UFH) inactivates free thrombin to inhibit platelet activation. Dosing should be per a weight-based protocol with serial partial thromboplastin time (PTT) monitoring. UFH is preferred if surgical intervention is expected within 24 hours due to the short half-life and easy reversal of effect with protamine sulfate.

Low-molecular-weight heparin (LMWH) has been shown to be as safe and effective in management of UA/NSTEMI as UFH. Additionally, LMWH has an easier dosing regimen than UFH and no routine aPTT monitoring is required. LMWH is renally cleared and renal dysfunction is a relative contraindication due to increased major bleeding. The degree of anticoagulation can be assessed by measurement of anti-Xa levels, although in clinical practice this is rarely performed. LMWH should be discontinued 24 hours prior to surgical intervention and replaced with UFH due to the long half-life of LMWH. LMWH should be initiated with a 30 mg intravenous loading dose followed by 1 mg/kg subcutaneous injection every 12 hours.

Direct thrombin inhibitors (DTI) inactivate both free and bound thrombin to inhibit platelet activation. There are three predominant DTIs: hirudin, bivalirudin, and argatroban.

Bivalirudin is the preferred DTI for periprocedural use in PCI with a short half-life (25 minutes) and a safety profile equivalent to UFH (hepatic, renal, and proteolytic clearance).

Hirudin and argatroban are FDA approved for use in heparin-induced thrombocytopenia. Hirudin is contraindicated in renal dysfunction due to primarily renal clearance. Argatroban has hepatic clearance and is suitable for patients with renal dysfunction.

Other Medications

Angiotensin-converting enzyme (ACE) inhibitors decrease morbidity/mortality particularly in ACS patients with diabetes or left-ventricular (LV) dysfunction. They are also thought to play a role in ventricular remodeling post-MI and should be initiated within 24 hours after presentation.

HMG-CoA reductase inhibitors (statins) may have pleiotropic effects, and in addition to lipid lowering, they are thought to play a role in attenuating the inflammatory cascade. In the MIRACL trial, atorvastatin 80 mg daily was associated with a significant reduction in death, nonfatal MI, resuscitated cardiac arrest or recurrent severe ischemia (17.4% to 14.8%). Based on this finding we preferentially initiate lipid-lowering therapy with atorvastatin 80 mg daily in patients under 70 years of age (40 mg atorvastatin for >70 years old).

Fibrinolytics are contraindicated in the treatment of NSTEMI and have proven harm in this setting.

SURGICAL MANAGEMENT

Coronary Angiography and Percutaneous Intervention

Early Intervention Versus Conservative Management

Multiple studies have demonstrated a clear benefit to an early invasive strategy compared to a conservative approach in medium- to high-risk patients (elevated troponin, ST-segment deviation, or TIMI risk score ≥3). Early invasive therapy involves coronary angiography and revascularization within 48 hours of symptom onset. In a conservative therapy approach, best reserved for low-risk patients, coronary angiography is performed only for patients with recurrent ischemic pain or a strongly positive stress test.

Drug-eluting stents (DES) have become the predominant choice for percutaneous intervention due to decreased rates of in-stent restenosis. However, questions have been raised as to whether the rate of catastrophic very late (>1 year after the index procedure) stent thrombosis may be increased with the use of DES. Currently, there are no consensus guidelines available to guide the use of DES in the setting of acute myocardial infarction and further studies are needed.

DISCHARGE

In our institution patients with NSTEMI who are hemodynamically stable do not typically require cardiac intensive care unit (CICU). However, serial cardiac enzymes and ECG should be obtained while patients await angiography. Patients who are admitted to CICU should be started on oral medications as previously discussed. Patients with ongoing ischemia, particularly those with recurrent chest pain, should not be transferred to the regular nursing floor prior to resolution of this issue.

RECOMMENDED READING

1. Braunwald E, Antman EM, Beasley JW, et al. ACC/AHA 2002 guideline update for the management of patients with unstable angina and non-ST-Segment elevation myocardial infarction—summary. *J Am Coll Cardiol.* 2002; 40(7)1366–1374.
2. Ayala TH, Schulman SP, Pathogenesis and early management of non-ST-segment elevation acute coronary syndromes. *Cardiol Clin.* 2006; (24)19–35.
3. Bavry AA, Kumbhani DJ, Rassi AN, et al. Benefit of early invasive therapy in acute coronary syndromes: a meta-analysis of contemporary randomized clinical trials. *J Am Coll Cardiol.* 2006; (28) 1319–1325.

Mechanical Complications of Acute Myocardial Infarction

SAIF ANWARUDDIN

Mechanical complications of acute myocardial infarction are distinct clinical syndromes. A high degree of suspicion in the postmyocardial infarction period must be maintained for accurate diagnosis. Early recognition of these complications and timely management can lead to significantly improved outcomes.

This chapter will cover acute mitral regurgitation, ventricular septal rupture, left-ventricular free-wall rupture, and left-ventricular (LV) failure. In the acute setting, the mainstays of diagnosing these entities include the physical exam, echocardiography, right-heart catheterization, and angiography.

ACUTE MITRAL REGURGITATION

Mitral regurgitation in the postmyocardial-infarction setting is often associated with partial or complete rupture of the papillary muscle. Mitral regurgitation can also result from annular dilation due to left ventricular dilation. Regardless of etiology, the presence of mitral regurgitation is a poor prognostic factor. For this discussion, we will focus on acute mitral regurgitation caused by acute papillary muscle rupture.

Acute papillary muscle results from acute cessation of blood flow to the posterior descending artery (most commonly coming off the right coronary artery). The anterior papillary muscle receives dual blood supply from both the left anterior descending artery and the left circumflex artery, so it is typically protected against acute rupture. The incidence of papillary muscle rupture complicating acute myocardial infarction is estimated to be 1%. According to data from the SHOCK Trial Registry, patients are more likely to be female and less likely to have ST-segment elevation at presentation.

VENTRICULAR SEPTAL RUPTURE

Ventricular septal rupture (VSR) is a well-defined complication of myocardial infarction that portends a poor prognosis. The incidence is lower in the era of fibrinolytics and emergency percutaneous coronary revascularization. The SHOCK Trial Registry reported that 55 patients of 939 presenting with cardiogenic shock had VSR as an etiology. It typically occurs in massive myocardial infarction involving either the left-anterior descending artery or the right-coronary-artery territories.

LEFT-VENTRICULAR FREE-WALL RUPTURE

Free-wall rupture is typically a complication of ST-segment elevation myocardial infarctions. The incidence is 2.7% in patients with postmyocardial infarction shock, but true event rate is difficult to ascertain as it is typically a catastrophic occurrence. Notably, these patients typically did not have diabetes, extensive peripheral vascular disease, or prior myocardial infarctions. It presents more commonly in the anterior wall from left-anterior descending or left-circumflex-artery territory infarcts in female and elderly patients. The presentation can vary from asymptomatic to sudden cardiovascular death, depending on the extent of rupture and whether or not it remains contained.

LEFT-VENTRICULAR PUMP FAILURE

Pump failure is the most common etiology for cardiogenic shock in the setting of myocardial infarction. The presentation is often quite dramatic and implies significant underlying coronary-artery disease in multiple territories. There are clinical (Killip) and invasive (Forrester) methods of classifying the degree of pump failure. Pump failure may result in patients with ST or non-ST-elevation myocardial infarctions. Risk factors for pump failure include age, diabetes mellitus, and 3-vessel disease. It is important to exclude the previously mentioned mechanical complications in the evaluation of patients presenting with cardiogenic shock.

ACUTE MANAGEMENT

Diagnostic Tests:

- **ECG:**
  - ST elevation in the inferior leads or ST depression in V1 and V2 suggestive of posterior myocardial infarction are more common in acute papillary muscle rupture.
  - Anterior ST elevation may suggest ventricular septal rupture, free-wall rupture, or pump failure
  - Conduction abnormalities are common in ventricular septal rupture.
- **CXR:** Check for pulmonary edema.
- **Transthoracic Echocardiography:**
  - Evaluate for left-ventricular function in multiple orthogonal views.
  - If there is valvular regurgitation, the etiology should be defined.
  - Place color-flow Doppler across the ventricular septum in the parasternal, apical four chamber and subcostal views.
  - Consider TEE if unable to characterize the valvular regurgitation or if there is a high suspicion of a mechanical complication not characterized on TTE.
- **Right-Heart Catheterization:**
  - Look for large V waves on pulmonary capillary wedge pressure tracing and an elevated pulmonary arterial oxygen saturation to rule out acute mitral regurgitation
  - Send proximal and distal arterial saturations or perform a shunt run to evaluate for ventricular septal rupture.
  - Evaluate for diastolic equalization of pressures to rule out tamponade if there is free-wall rupture.

Management:

- **Tools:** at least two large-bore IV lines
- **STAT labs:** CBC, CMP, PT/PTT, type and screen
- **Therapies:**
  - Initiate therapy for ST or NSTEMI as documented in previous chapters.
  - Diuretics are often indicated due to pulmonary edema resulting from left-ventricular failure.
  - IV Nitroglycerin for chest discomfort or ischemic symptoms.

- – Sodium Nitroprusside: aggressive afterload reduction is necessary to improve forward flow if the blood pressure can tolerate.
- – Vasopressor therapy with norepinephrine may be necessary if hypotension is extreme.
- – Intra-aortic balloon pump: should be implemented in patients with shock as quickly as possible.
- – Left-heart catheterization: should be performed to delineate coronary anatomy.

Surgical: Patients with a confirmed diagnosis of papillary muscle rupture, ventricular septal rupture, or free-wall rupture require immediate surgical evaluation.

CCU Tip: A high suspicion of a mechanical complication post-myocardial infarction is necessary for prompt diagnosis and therapy. Bedside echo and/or right-heart catheterization may be performed quickly and will help direct therapy.

CLINICAL PRESENTATION

The clinical presentation of these four complications can range from asymptomatic to fulminant cardiogenic shock thus requiring a high level of suspicion to enable a timely diagnosis:

- Recurrent chest pain
- Hemodynamic collapse/cardiogenic shock
- Respiratory distress
- Syncope
- Sudden cardiac death
- Symptoms of low cardiac output (i.e., altered mental status, renal failure, cool extremities)
- Unremitting nausea (may be more suggestive of free-wall rupture)

PHYSICAL EXAMINATION

Patients with a postinfarction mechanical complication often present with the typical signs of cardiogenic shock such as tachycardia, hypotension, cool extremities, and mental-status changes. In addition, patients with papillary muscle rupture develop a harsh pansystolic murmur at the apex that radiates to the axilla. Patients with ventricular septal rupture or free-wall rupture can also develop a new murmur usually at the left sternal border and may also have a new pericardial friction rub.

DIAGNOSTIC TESTS

ECG with ST changes consistent with an inferior or posterior infarction may be more suggestive of acute papillary muscle rupture. Anterior ST elevation myocardial infarction more often predisposes to free-wall rupture and pump failure. Conduction abnormalities may be seen with ventricular septal rupture.

Chest x-ray will demonstrate pulmonary edema.

Transthoracic echocardiography (TTE) is the primary diagnostic modality to identify papillary muscle rupture or flail mitral leaflet. Color-flow imaging is helpful in quantifying the degree of mitral regurgitation and excluding other possible etiologies such as LV failure or ventricular septal rupture. If free-wall rupture is diagnosed, echo can evaluate the extent of free-wall rupture and determine whether it is contained (pseudoaneurysm). Furthermore, echocardiography can be used to establish the presence of cardiac tamponade. If unable to visualize the free-wall rupture, contrast can be used to demonstrate extravasation into the pericardial space (Fig. 4.1).

Right-heart catheterization should reveal large V waves in acute severe mitral regurgitation. These can also be seen in ventricular septal rupture (Fig. 4.2), so a shunt run or proximal and distal-arterial-saturation samples should be obtained to differentiate the two. Typically, an 8% or

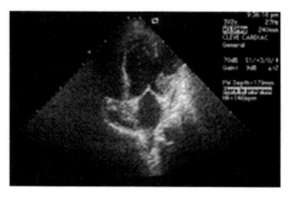

FIGURE 4.1. Free-wall rupture as seen on 2-D transthoracic echocardiography.

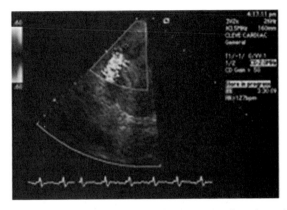

FIGURE 4.2. Doppler echocardiography demonstrates flow through a post-myocardial ventricular septal rupture.

greater increase in the oxygen saturations in either the right ventricle (RV) or pulmonary-artery circulation is noted. For patients with LV pump failure, the right-heart catheter can assist in the titration of medical therapy and help define the etiology of the hypotension (i.e., cardiogenic vs. septic or hypovolemic). Fluoroscopic guidance is ideal to ensure proper catheter placement especially in the setting of possible VSR.

Left-heart catheterization will not only define the coronary anatomy, but ventriculography can quantitatively assess for both mitral regurgitation and a ventricular septal rupture.

MEDICAL MANAGEMENT

Early recognition of a mechanical complication is necessary for treatment and emergent surgical intervention. There is a high mortality associated with these entities, but positive outcomes are possible with aggressive diagnostic testing and therapy.

Afterload Reduction

After the diagnosis has been established, the first step is to introduce afterload reduction in the form of intravenous nitroglycerin and nitroprusside as hemodynamic parameters allow. The goal should be to achieve mean arterial pressures of 60 to 65 mmHg. Nitroglycerin should be preferentially titrated initially to prevent coronary steal. An intra-aortic balloon pump may also be utilized to reduce afterload especially in the setting of a ventricular septal rupture as it decreases flow across the shunt.

Vasopressor Therapy

Pharmacologic afterload reduction may be contraindicated in patients with mechanical complications postmyocardial infarction due to severe hypotension. Thus, these patients will often require vasopressor therapy. Norepinephrine may be necessary to maintain an adequate perfusion pressure and can be used in conjunction with an intra-aortic balloon pump to maintain a mean arterial pressure between 60 to 65 mmHg.

Diuresis

Diuretic therapy with furosemide is often necessary to relieve pulmonary edema. Because these patients are often in cardiogenic shock and have poor renal perfusion, hemodynamically guided diuresis can be useful in optimizing a patient's fluid status.

SURGICAL MANAGEMENT

Acute papillary muscle rupture, ventricular septal rupture, and free-wall rupture usually cannot be treated medically for a prolonged duration, so prompt surgical consultation is necessary to prevent excess mortality. The goal of CCU care is to stabilize these patients, which may not always be possible. The best outcomes depend on early surgical intervention as even apparently stable patients often deteriorate rapidly and unexpectedly.

RECOMMENDED READING

1. Topol EJ. *Textbook of Cardiovascular Medicine*, 3rd ed. Philadelphia, PA: Lippincott Williams & Wilkins, 2007.
2. Griffin BP, Topol EJ. *Manual of Cardiovascular Medicine*, 2nd ed. Philadelphia, PA: Lippincott Williams & Wilkins, 2004.
3. Thompson CR, Buller CE, Sleeper LA, et al. Cardiogenic shock due to acute severe mitral regurgitation complicating acute myocardial infarction: a report from the SHOCK Trial Registry. *JACC.* 2000; (36):1104–1109.
4. Slater J, Brown RJ, Antonelli TA, et al. Cardiogenic shock due to cardiac free-wall rupture or tamponade after acute myocardial infarction: a report from the SHOCK Trial Registry. *JACC.* 2000; (36):1117–1122.
5. Menon V, Webb JG, Hillis D, et al. Outcome and profile of ventricular septal rupture with cardiogenic shock after myocardial infarction: a report from the SHOCK Trial Registry. *JACC.* 2000; (36):1110–1116.
6. Webb JG, Sleeper LA, Buller CE, et al. Implications of the timing of onset of cardiogenic shock after acute myocardial infarction: a report from the SHOCK Trial Registry. *JACC.* 2000; (36): 1084–1090.
7. Holmes DR, Berger PB, Granger CB, et al. Cardiogenic shock in patients with acute ischemic syndromes and without ST-segment elevation. *Circulation.* 1999; (100): 2067–2073.

CHAPTER 5

Right-Ventricular Infarction

JOHN M. GALLA

Right-ventricular (RV) infarction can occur in up to 50% of inferior myocardial infarctions (MI), usually due to an occlusion of the right coronary artery proximal to the RV marginal branch. While mild RV prognosis in the setting dysfunction after inferior or inferoposterior wall MI is common, significant RV failure occurs in only 10% of patients. RV infarction carries a poor short-term prognosis in the setting of acute coronary syndrome (ACS); however, RV is thin walled, requires less oxygen, and has blood flow that occurs in both systole and diastole; thus most patients who survive to discharge typically experience complete recovery over time.

PRESENTATION

Patients with RV infarction typically present with the triad of hypotension, elevated jugular venous distention (JVD), and absence of dyspnea. Severe RV failure is associated with diaphoresis, cold and clammy extremities, renal failure, and altered mental status secondary to low cardiac output. Kussmaul's sign (inspiratory increase in jugular venous pressure) may be observed.

PHYSICAL EXAMINATION

- Hypotension
- Elevated jugular venous distention (JVP)
- Clear lung fields
- Pulsus paradoxus (Diminished systolic pressure with inspiration)
- Kussmaul's sign (Failure of JVP to decrease with inspiration)

43

ACUTE MANAGEMENT

Diagnostic Tests:

- **ECG:** Likely to show inferior (II, III, aVF) ST elevation, right-sided leads (mirror image of left-sided leads) with ST elevation, especially V4R. A clue on the standard 12-lead ECG is ST elevation in lead V1 in the setting of an inferior STEMI.
- **Echo:** Evaluate ventricular function, right-ventricular dilatation, right-atrial enlargement; assess tricuspid regurgitation and right-ventricular systolic pressure.
- **Pulmonary artery (PA) catheter:** Assess right-sided filling pressures, pulmonary capillary wedge pressure. Usually high right-sided pressures with a low pulmonary capillary wedge pressure. Right-atrial pressure >10 mmHg and within 5 mmHg of pulmonary capillary wedge pressure (or greater) is suggestive of right-ventricle infarct.

Management:

- Activate cath lab, place urinary drainage catheter, shave both groins
- **Tools:** Arterial line, two large bore IVs, portable CXR
- **STAT labs:** CMP, CBC, PT, INR, aPTT, Cardiac Enzymes, Lipids, HbA1C, BNP, CRP
- **Meds:**
  - Aspirin 81 mg × 4 by mouth
  - Heparin weight-based bolus + drip
  - Antiplatelet therapy as indicated in Chapter 2
  - IV isotonic saline to maintain right-sided filling pressure
- Consider dobutamine if fluids are ineffective at maintaining blood pressure
- Consider IABP in hypotensive patients with concomitant left-ventricular dysfunction
- Consider temporary atrioventricular sequential pacing with an atrioventricular delay of 200 mseconds in patients with heart block

Surgical:

- Immediate coronary intervention for STEMI
- Right-ventricular assist device is indicated in the care of patients who remain in cardiogenic shock

> **CCU Tip:** Hemodynamic monitoring is crucial; Avoid nitroglycerine, beta blockers, angiotensin converting enzymes inhibitors, narcotics, and diuretics.
>
> **Acute Management**
>
> **Diagnostic Tests:**
>
> - **ECG:** Evaluate for ST changes, deep symmetrical prechordial T-wave inversions, atrioventricular block, arrhythmias; repeat serially and especially with changes in chest pain
> - **TTE:** Evaluate left- and right-ventricular function, wall-motion abnormalities, pericardial effusions, septal defects, aortic root dissection, and valvular regurgitation (especially mitral insufficiency)

DIFFERENTIAL DIAGNOSIS

- Pulmonary embolism
- Pericardial effusion
- Constrictive pericarditis
- Aortic dissection

RISK FACTORS

- RV hypertrophy
- Traditional risk factors for coronary atherosclerosis
- Location of mitral insufficiency (MI)

DIAGNOSTIC TESTS

Electrocardiogram (ECG) is the first diagnostic test to be performed. Depending on the availability of a cardiac catheterization laboratory at the presenting facility, patients should be transferred to a facility with a catheterization laboratory or receive fibrinolysis. Adjunctive testing should not delay reperfusion. For patients awaiting reperfusion, echocardiography may be used to confirm RV infarction physiology. In patients who remain hypotensive after intravenous fluids and require intravenous vasopressors, pulmonary artery catheterization should be considered.

ECG performed with standard left-sided precordial leads usually shows inferior (leads II, III, aVF; Fig. 5.1) or posterior (deep S wave in

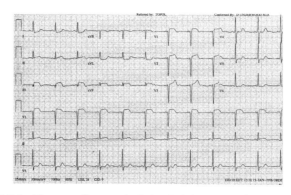

FIGURE 5.1. Electrocardiogram depicting inferior myocardial infarction with RV involvement.

V1, V2 with ST-segment depression) ST-segment elevation myocardial infarction. With leads V_1R-V_6R across the right precordium, there is typically ST-segment elevation of greater than 1.0 mm in V_4R, but may be seen in leads $V_{3-6}R$ (Fig. 5.2). Right bundle branch and high-grade atrioventricular block are also common.

Echocardiography is useful for quantifying RV function and assessing right-sided filling pressures. RV wall-motion abnormalities are typically seen in addition to septal dyskinesis. RV dilatation and right-atrial enlargement are also key findings to support RV infarction physiology.

A **pulmonary artery catheter** can be an invaluable tool for difficult-to-manage patients. An accurate assessment of pulmonary artery and

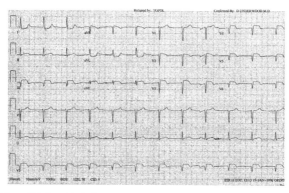

FIGURE 5.2. Right-sided electrocardiogram demonstrating RV infarction with ST elevation in V4.

pulmonary capillary wedge pressure (PCWP) can confirm the presence of RV infarct physiology, guide fluid administration, and be used to time the initiation and titration of inotropes. Right-atrial pressure in patients with RV infarction is usually greater than 10 mmHg and also greater than 80% of PCWP. A PA catheter should be placed with care as induction or worsening of arrhythmia is possible, which may precipitate or worsen hypotension.

MEDICAL MANAGEMENT

Patients presenting with symptoms consistent with an acute coronary syndrome and ST-segment elevation should be referred for immediate reperfusion therapy (cardiac catheterization or fibrinolysis). Patients should be examined for evidence of RV and/or left-ventricular (LV) dysfunction. Right-sided ECG leads are helpful to confirm evidence of RV involvement.

Patients should receive two large-bore intravenous lines and if awaiting cardiac catheterization, should have both groins shaved and a urinary-drainage catheter placed.

In patients with evidence of RV infarction, initial medical management should include supplemental oxygen by nasal cannula and aspirin 81 mg × 4 chewed. **Avoid nitrates, narcotics, diuretics, ACE inhibitors, and beta blockers** as these patients are extremely sensitive to reductions in preload, and these agents may precipitate an exaggerated hypotensive response.

Intravenous heparin should be started as a weight-based bolus and drip to maintain the activated partial thromboplastin time between 42 to 56 seconds.

For hypotensive patients, volume expansion with isotonic saline should be administered to maintain preload. This may require several liters of fluid. Use PA catheter to guide fluid management in these patients.

If initial attempts at volume resuscitation fail to maintain adequate blood pressure, inotropic support should be initiated. Dobutamine is the initial agent of choice and is typically started at a 5 µg/kg/min infusion rate. Titrate dobutamine and use additional agents as necessary to maintain adequate perfusion pressure.

For patients presenting with high-grade heart block or bradyarrhythmias, atrioventricular (AV) sequential pacing has been shown to significantly improve hemodynamic function in patients with hypotension refractory to volume resuscitation.

In hypotensive patients with concomitant LV dysfunction, afterload reduction with sodium nitroprusside or an intra-aortic balloon pump may be warranted. However, sodium nitroprusside should be used with extreme caution in the first 24 hours of a STEMI.

CLINICAL PRESENTATION TIPS

- Hypotension: Suspect right ventricle under filling, continue IV fluids
- Respiratory distress: Acute heart failure due to fluid resuscitation, if a late presentation may be due to pulmonary embolism
- Bradycardia: May be due to sinus or atrioventricular-node dysfunction due to disruption of nodal blood supply or to the associated vagotonia related to inferior MI
- ↓urine output: Low cardiac output
- Post PCI chest pain: Consider pericarditis

COMPLICATIONS

Shock due to unrecognized RV infarction is common. Avoid reflex (inappropriate) use of vasodilators in RV infarct.

Arrhythmias are common in patients presenting with RV infarction due to interruption of blood supply to important cardiac pacing structures. High-degree or complete AV block has been reported in up to half of RV infarct patients and is frequently accompanied by bradycardia and resultant hypotension. Atrial fibrillation occurs in up to one third of patients and may be a result of atrial infarction or dilation from volume overload.

Ventricular septal rupture may occur if transmural RV septal infarction is present. If abnormally high right-sided pressures are needed to maintain adequate RV preload, flow through a ventricular septal defect or patent foramen ovale may produce a right-to-left shunt with resultant hypoxia.

RV thrombus with resultant **pulmonary embolism** is possible in cases of severe RV dysfunction.

Pericarditis is common following RV infarction due to the relatively thin dimensions of the normal right ventricle, thus increasing the likelihood of transmural infarction.

DISCHARGE

Patient with RV infarct should remain in the intensive care unit (ICU) until a stable hemodynamic status is reached. Severe cases of RV infarction may require up to 10 to 14 days of ICU stay. Almost all cases of RV infarction improve with time. Therefore, patience and invasive hemodynamic monitoring are necessary to prepare patients for discharge. Once hemodynamically stable, a low dose of ACE inhibitors may be considered. All patients should be on a stable oral dose of medications to maintain blood pressure and heart rate before leaving the cardiac intensive care unit (CICU).

RECOMMENDED READING

1. Antman EM, Anbe DT, Armstrong PW, et al. ACC/AHA guidelines for the management of patients with ST-elevation myocardial infarction; A report of the American College of Cardiology/American Heart Association Task Force on Practice Guidelines (Committee to Revise the 1999 Guidelines for the management of patients with acute myocardial infarction). *J Am Coll Cardiol.* 2004; 44:E1–E211.
2. Tschopp D, Mukherjee D. Complications of myocardial infarction. In: Griffin BP, Topol EJ, eds. *Manual of Cardiovascular Medicine.* Philadelphia: Lippincott Williams & Wilkins; 2004:3–26.
3. O'Rourke RA, Dell'Italia LJ. Diagnosis and management of right ventricular myocardial infarction. *Curr Probl Cardiol.* 2004; 29(1):6–47.

CHAPTER **6**

Post-Coronary Intervention Management

THOMAS H. WANG

Patients who are postcoronary intervention require specialized monitoring with staff sensitive to the unique aspects of their care.

PRESENTATION

These patients present after a coronary intervention usually in an intensive care unit (ICU) setting or in a step-down unit. Complications that occur after an intervention may present surreptitiously and should be evaluated quickly.

DIFFERENTIAL DIAGNOSIS

- Access site complication: arteriovenous (AV) fistula, retroperitoneal bleed, pseudoaneurysm
- Cardiac tamponade
- Contrast nephropathy
- Vasovagal reaction
- Arrhythmias
- Acute pulmonary edema or pulmonary hemorrhage if on IIb/IIIa inhibitor
- Cardiogenic shock
- Stroke
- Dissection
- Stent thrombosis

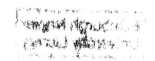

ACUTE MANAGEMENT

Diagnostic Tests:

- Physical exam: obtain a baseline blood pressure and heart rate, evaluate vascular access sites for hematoma and bruits, check distal extremity perfusion, check the patient's flank for signs of retroperitoneal bleeding.
- ECG: a stat ECG should be ordered in patients with chest pain or shortness of breath after a PCI has been performed. Serial ECGs are necessary in patients with a peri-procedural increase in cardiac enzymes.
- Angiography: review the films to evaluate if a procedural complications such as coronary dissection or distal perforation occurred but was unrecognized in the catheterization laboratory or if femoral arterial access was obtained too high or too low.
- Ultrasound: check vascular studies of the access site to rule out hematoma, arteriovenous fistula, or pseudoaneurysm formation.
- Transthoracic echo: should be utilized to rule out a pericardial effusion, new wall-motion abnormalities, or the development of a shunt
- CT scan: should be emergently obtained if there are mental-status changes and/or physical exam findings consistent with stroke

Management:

- **Tools:** rarely may need Swan-Ganz catheter for hemodynamic management
- **STAT labs:** CBC, CMP, PT, INR, PTT, type and screen, cardiac enzymes repeated three times every 8 hours

Medications (depending on the etiology of the complication)

- Consider blood transfusions for an access site complication or bleed
- Platelet transfusions may be utilized for severe bleeding or GP IIb/IIIa induced bleeding—except in patients who have received small molecule IIb/IIIa inhibitors
- Atropine should be readily available for a vasovagal induced bradycardic episode

- Consider alternative anticoagulation for patients with HIT
  - Lepirudin (recombinant hirudin) at IV loading dose of 0.4 mg/kg over 15-20 seconds with a maintenance infusion of 0.15 mg/kg/hr. Avoid in patients with CKD
  - Argatroban at 2 µg/kg/min infusion (maximum 10 µg/kg/min). Avoid in patients with hepatic dysfunction
  - Bivalirudin with a 1.75 mg/kg/hr or at 1.00 mg/kg/hr in patients with a creatinine clearance <30 mL/min or 0.25 mg/kg/hr in patients on dialysis

Surgical: May require surgical repair for femoral artery to stop bleeding.

CCU Tip: Any patients with retroperitoneal bleeding should be admitted to the coronary care unit and monitored closely. Have a very low threshold for vascular surgery consultation.

DIAGNOSTIC TESTS

ECGs should be serially ordered in post-coronary intervention (PCI) patients to assess for new conduction abnormalities and in patients with recurrent chest pain to assess for abrupt vessel closure or stent thrombosis.

CXR is necessary in patients with respiratory distress especially in the context of thrombocytopenia, hemoptysis, and IIB/IIA inhibitor use, which could suggest pulmonary hemorrhage. Additionally, the clinical diagnosis of pulmonary edema and/or aspiration pneumonia may be supported.

Ultrasound may be utilized to evaluate for an access site complication such as an AV fistula, hematoma, or pseudoaneurysm. A retroperitoneal bleed may often be diagnosed clinically, and a CT scan may not be indicated, especially if the patient is unstable.

Transthoracic echocardiography can quickly and accurately diagnose cardiac tamponade (Chapter 18).

Head CT is very helpful to rule out a stroke in patients with mental-status changes. An MRI/A may be necessary as well.

CLINICAL PRESENTATION TIPS

a. **Chest pain** can be due to abrupt vessel closure (i.e., dissection), periprocedural myocardial infarction, stent thrombosis, and postcoronary intervention pain. Most chest pain after coronary intervention, however, is NOT related to coronary ischemia. Repeat coronary angiography is rarely indicated in patients with chest pain that is not accompanied by electrocardiographic changes or hemodynamic instability.

b. **Hypotension** may be due to hypovolemia, vasovagal reaction, cardiac tamponade, or retroperitoneal bleeding from the arterial access site.

c. **Diminished pulse** is often the first presentation of a dissected vascular access site or thrombotic occlusion of the access site.

d. **Shortness of breath** is often an expression of pulmonary edema due to contrast or ischemia. Pulmonary hemorrhage should also be considered in the context of antiplatelet therapy.

e. **Mental-status change** should prompt an evaluation for a transient ischemic attack or stroke (embolic or hemorrhagic).

f. **Decreased urine output** may be caused by contrast nephropathy or cholesterol emboli, but is most commonly related to intravascular depletion due to contrast-induced osmotic diuresis, prolonged nothing by mouth status, and possibly blood loss.

g. **Groin/back pain** can be due to retroperitoneal bleeding or presence of a pseudoaneurysm.

MEDICAL MANAGEMENT

Arterial access complications include retroperitoneal bleeding, pseudoaneurysm formation, arteriovenous fistula formation, and arterial thrombosis or dissection. A retroperitoneal bleed or hematoma is often associated with a high femoral arterial puncture site while a pseudoaneurysm is associated with a low femoral arterial puncture. Complications are more common in the obese, elderly, critically ill, and in patients on increasing anticoagulation. Additionally, the size of the sheath and frequency of vascular access can predispose to a vascular complication.

Thrombotic occlusion of the artery requires an emergent vascular surgery consultation.

Arteriovenous fistula may require surgical repair.

Arterial pseudoaneurysms are detected by the presence of a pulsatile mass with a systolic bruit over the catheter insertion site. Small pseudo-

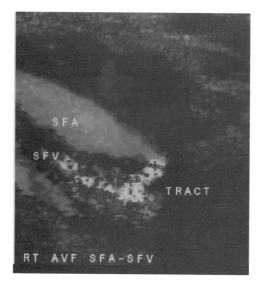

FIGURE 6.1. Right superficial femoral artery to vein fistula Doppler ultrasound.

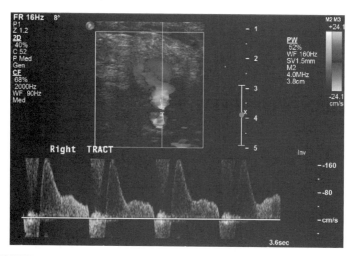

FIGURE 6.2. Right superficial femoral artery pseudoaneurysm Doppler ultrasound.

aneurysms can be treated with ultrasound guided injection of thrombin. However, those that are larger may require surgical treatment.

Periprocedural myocardial infarction is characterized by a threefold increase in the CK-MB level from baseline. This can be due to a number of intraprocedural complications such as side-branch compromise, hypotension, thrombus formation, coronary dissection, or the use of atherectomy devices. Patients with large periprocedural infarctions, that is those with CK-MB increase of more than 5 to 10 times baseline, appear to be at increased risk for late cardiac death.

Abrupt vessel closure is a feared complication that typically occurs in the catheterization laboratory but can also occur within hours after the angioplasty. It is usually unheralded, but can be associated with discontinuation of anticoagulation, platelet transfusion, and hypotension. The incidence of abrupt vessel closure is much less with stents than with balloon angioplasty, but can still occur in high-risk patients. Reviewing the angiograms can be useful to determine predisposing factors such as a residual dissection, suboptimal postintervention coronary flow, and degree of preintervention plaque burden. Patients with chest pain and ECG changes indicative of abrupt closure should undergo repeat catheterization and receive optimal antiplatelet therapy including heparin, clopidogrel, and a glycoprotein IIb/IIIa inhibitor.

A stroke may present with an altered mental status and/or sensory or motor symptoms. There should be a low threshold for a neurologic exam or consultation and a head CT. CVAs may occur either because of hemorrhage or embolization.

Arrhythmias often occur postprocedurally. Most commonly, vasovagal reactions may be seen with transient bradycardia and hypotension with associated nausea and diaphoresis. These reactions may be seen in conjunction with increased groin pressure, pain, anxiety, and hypovolemia. Additionally, conduction abnormalities may be noted if a septal branch perforator is compromised during an intervention.

Renal failure may be seen in patients with preexisting renal disease or if excess contrast is utilized. This is avoided by minimizing the use of contrast during the procedure itself as well as providing hydration and utilizing a low-osmolar contrast agent. Additionally, N-acetylcysteine may be utilized (600 mg twice daily). Occasionally, acute renal failure may occur secondary to atheroembolism.

Pulmonary hemorrhage may occur with patients who have received IIb/IIIa inhibitors. These agents need to be discontinued immediately in these patients. Mechanical ventilation may be necessary and frequent CBCs checked to consider platelet or blood transfusions.

Cardiac tamponade may occur due to coronary-artery dissection or perforation and should be considered in patients who have developed sudden hypotension, tachycardia, and/or respiratory distress. An echo should be done rapidly to rule out this complication (Chapter 18).

Thrombocytopenia is quite common in patients who are postcardiac catheterization, but a severe and sustained drop in platelet counts should raise the suspicion for heparin-induced thrombocytopenia—especially if the patient has prior exposure to heparin. This can be diagnosed by checking a HIT assay and platelet factor 4 antibodies. Additionally, glycoprotein IIb/IIIa induced thrombocytopenia especially from abciximab is a well-described phenomenon and must be carefully monitored for.

Distal ischemic complications may also occur as a result of atheroemboli; however, this is very rare. Prompt removal of the arterial sheath and appropriate anticoagulation are important to prevent this complication.

Infection is rare but can occur. The most common organisms are staphylococcus aureus, coagulase-negative staphylococcus, and group B streptococcus. Risk factors include duration of the procedure, the number of catheterizations at the same access site, difficult vascular access, and arterial sheath in place for more than 1 day.

RECOMMENDED READING

1. Lincoff AM. Abupt vessel closure. In: Topol, EJ, ed. *Textbook of Interventional Cardiology*. 4th ed. Philadelphia: Elsevier; 2003:267–278.
2. Baim DS, Simon DI. Complications and optimal use of adjunctive pharmacology. In: Baim DS, ed. *Cardiac Catheterization, Angiography, and Intervention*. 7th ed. Philadelphia: Lippincott Williams & Wilkins; 2006: 36–71.

Acute Decompensated Valvular Heart Disease

CHAPTER 7

Decompensated Aortic Stenosis

MEHDI H. SHISHEHBOR

Decompensated aortic stenosis (AS) results from progressive obstruction of the aortic valve associated with congestive heart failure, angina, or recurrent syncope. The main causes of native valve AS are congenital, calcific, and rheumatic. (Prosthetic valve stenosis is discussed separately.) The normal aortic valve area is 3 to 4 cm^2; however, in severe AS this area is frequently less than 1 cm^2. Decompensated AS can present in the setting of preserved or diminished left-ventricular (LV) function.

PRESENTATION

Patients with AS can present with angina (50% 5-year survival rate without surgery), syncope (50% 3-year survival rate without surgery), and heart failure. As AS progresses patients typically present with exertional dyspnea, orthopnea, syncope, chest pain, or paroxysmal nocturnal dyspnea (mean survival time of less than 2 years). Patients commonly present to cardiac intensive care unit (CICU) with signs and symptoms of heart failure, hypotension, cardiogenic shock, or arrhythmias.

PHYSICAL EXAMINATION

- Systolic ejection murmur
- Severe AS is associated with long murmur that peaks late in systole
- Diminished aortic component of S_2
- S_3 and/or S_4
- Pulsus parvus et tardus (low amplitude and late-peaking pulse)
- Brachial-radial delay

ACUTE MANAGEMENT

Diagnostic Tests:

- **TTE:** To diagnose aortic stenosis, determine the cause and severity, and assess left-ventricular function

Management:

- **Tools:** Arterial line, two large-bore IV lines, possibly Swan-Ganz catheter
- **STAT labs:** type and cross, CBC, CMP, PT, INR, PTT, ECG, portable CXR, and cardiac enzymes

Medications:

- IV lasix to reach euvolemic state
- Sodium Nitroprusside if aortic stenosis associated with dilated moderate to severe left-ventricular dysfunction, avoid in patients with preserved left-ventricular function
- IABP if patient is hypotensive and cannot tolerate sodium nitroprusside
- If coronary artery disease (CAD) is present consider IV NTG (~40 µg/min) in conjunction with sodium nitroprusside

Surgical: Surgical consultation for aortic valve replacement. Consider percutaneous aortic valvuloplasty and possibly replacement if patient is a poor surgical candidate.

CCU Tip: Patient with dilated moderate to severe left-ventricular dysfunction significantly benefits from IV Nipride and/or IABP. Avoid any drug that can depress left-ventricular function such as Diprivan (propofol).

DIFFERENTIAL DIAGNOSIS

- Supravalvular AS: Associated with William's syndrome (mental retardation, short stature, renovascular hypertension, facial abnormalities, and hypercalcemia)
- Subvalvular AS: Fibromuscular membrane located in the LVOT
- Bicuspid AS: Associated with coarctation

- Unicuspid aortic valve
- Aortic pseudostenosis: Severe LV dysfunction with mild AS. The LV is unable to generate the appropriate force to open the small aortic valve

RISK FACTORS

- Age-related calcific degeneration
- Hypertension
- Smoking
- Hyperlipidemia
- Paget's disease
- End-stage renal disease (ESRD)
- Congenital bicuspid or unicuspid aortic valve

DIAGNOSTIC TESTS

Transthoracic echocardiography (TTE) should be at the bedside immediately upon patient's arrival to the intensive care unit (ICU). The parasternal long axis, two-dimensional and M-mode views are helpful to determine the etiology of AS, LV chamber dimensions, LV function, wall thickness, and presence of supra- and subvalvular aortic stenosis.

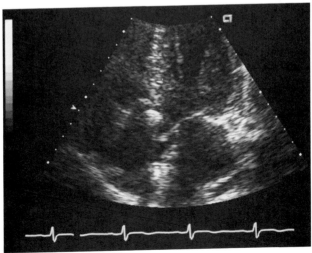

FIGURE 7.1. Severe aortic valve stenosis with moderate to severe calcification (white arrow).

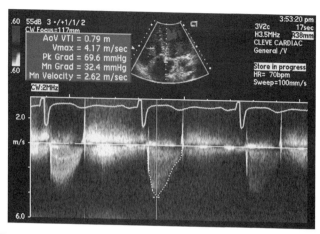

FIGURE 7.2. Continuous Doppler flow across the aortic valve on the same individual with peak and mean gradient of 69.6 mmHg and 32.4 mmHg, respectively.

Continuous-wave Doppler recording and pulse-wave Doppler in the apical five-chamber view are useful for the continuity equation. In addition, aortic regurgitation, coarctation, and wall-motion abnormalities should be evaluated.

Transesophageal echocardiography (TEE) can be used to better determine the etiology of aortic stenosis and obtain planimetry of the valve. However, in general, TTE is a better modality to determine aortic-valve gradients and area. TEE can also be used to diagnose subaortic stenosis and to differentiate it from hypertrophic cardiomyopathy. TEE can be done expeditiously at bedside.

Left-heart catheterization is indicated for almost all patients undergoing aortic-valve surgery. The risk associated with left-heart catheterization in patients with severe AS is around 0.2%. In addition, transaortic valvular gradient and aortic-valve area can be directly measured during cardiac catheterization if there are any concerns regarding the results from echocardiography. Severe AS is a relative contraindication to left ventriculography.

Right-heart catheterization is indicated for patients with severe AS and LV dysfunction who frequently require invasive monitoring to assess pulmonary capillary wedge pressure (PCWP) and cardiac output. In addition, right heart catheterization is helpful in guiding titration of medication such as lasix, IV nitroglycerin, and IV sodium nitroprusside.

MEDICAL MANAGEMENT

Initial physical exam should include a full cardiac and pulmonary exam to determine the degree of heart failure.

A minimum of two-large bore IV sites and a right heart catheter should be secured along with a radial arterial line and a type and screen sent with preliminary laboratory studies.

The goal in patients with severe decompensated AS is to maintain appropriate cardiac output while preventing volume overload and pulmonary edema. This is only a bridge for surgical or percutaneous intervention. Patients with preserved LV function rarely present with heart failure as the LV compensates for the fix obstruction. In these patients judicious use of intravenous (IV) lasix and IV Metoprolol 5 mg every 5 minutes for a goal heart rate of 70 to 80 should be sufficient. Decreasing the heart rate will increase the diastolic filling time and therefore may improve cardiac output. Avoid B-blockers in patients with low cardiac index.

Patients with severe AS and dilated LV require IV nipride in addition to IV lasix. In the presence of coronary artery disease (CAD) some experts recommend 40 to 50 µg/min of IV nitroglycerine to prevent coronary steal, which may be associated with nipride use. However, IV nitroglycerine should be used with care because of its venodilatory effects and its impact on preload. On occasion, patients with severe AS and LV dysfunction present with hypotension. These patients will benefit from IABP.

Patients with severe CAD and AS may also benefit from IABP if no contraindications to IABP are present. Ionotropes should be avoided in patients with fixed obstruction such as those with severe AS.

SURGICAL MANAGEMENT

Patients with severe decompensated AS require immediate surgical intervention once hemodynamically stable.

Occasionally, percutaneous aortic balloon valvuloplasty (PABV) may be used for palliative purposes or as a bridge to surgical correction. However, PABV has a short-term effect (typically <4 months) and may cause significant aortic insufficiency (AI). Patients with significant AI are not candidates for this procedure.

More recently, percutaneous aortic valve has been used in patients with severe to critical aortic stenosis who are not deemed surgical candidates.

CLINICAL PRESENTATION TIPS

- Hypotension: suspect severe left-ventricular dysfunction, acute myocardian infarction, dehydration, arrhythmias (e.g., atrial fibrillation)
- Angina: suspect coronary artery disease, severe aortic stenosis, arrhythmias (e.g., atrial fibrillation)
- Syncope: dehydration, acute myocardial infarction, arrhythmias (e.g., atrial fibrillation)
- Decreased urine output: low output state, dehydration/decrease preload

COMPLICATIONS

Syncope and Presyncope

Patients with AS are preload dependent. Initial step in evaluating patients with severe AS is to assess volume status. Careful volume replacement without overload is paramount.

Acute MI

CAD occurs in 40% to 80% of patients with angina and 25% to 30% of those without angina. Patients with an acute MI should be treated aggressively with invasive monitoring and IABP if indicated (low cardiac output, angina not relieved by optimum medications, and as a bridge to surgery).

Arrhythmias/Heart Block

These complications can have a profound impact on symptoms. As noted previously patients with severe/critical AS have very low reserve and are preload dependent. Any arrhythmia such as atrial fibrillation that impacts preload or increases oxygen demand will have a deleterious effects in these patients. Therefore, all arrhythmias should be treated aggressively. If hemodynamic compromise or end-organ damage is present cardioversion is the treatment of choice followed by appropriate IV drugs to prevent recurrence.

End-Organ Involvement

Severe/critical AS may be associated with low output state leading to syncope and renal insufficiency. Surgical intervention is the treatment of choice; however, in the acute setting attention should be given to preload, diastolic filling time, and afterload reduction in patients with moderate to severe LV dysfunction. Any underlying condition such as CAD or arrhythmias should be corrected.

DISCHARGE

Patients with decompensated aortic stenosis have a poor prognosis and require mechanical treatment of AS. We recommend that these patients remain in CICU until surgical or percutaneous decisions have been made. In patients with moderate AS, the underlying reason for their admission to CICU should be addressed. Typically, these patients should leave the CICU with beta blockers, statins, aspirin, and occasionally with ACE inhibitors if it can be tolerated.

RECOMMENDED READING

1. Khot UN, Novaro GM, Popovic ZB, et al. Nitroprusside in critically ill patients with left ventricular dysfunction and aortic stenosis. *N Engl J Med* 2003; 348:1756–1763.
2. Carabello BA, Stewart WJ, Crawford FA. Aortic valve disease. In Topol EJ, ed. *Textbook of Cardiovascular Medicine.* 2nd ed. Philadelphia: Lippincott-Raven, 2002:509–528.

CHAPTER 8

Acute Aortic Insufficiency

THOMAS H. WANG

A cute aortic insufficiency (AI) occurs due to either failure of leaflet coaptation, leaflet perforation or an abnormal aortic root that distorts the aortic cusps. It is typically due to chest-wall trauma, endocarditis, or aortic dissection. Unlike chronic AI, the left ventricle is unable to compensate for the rapid hemodynamic changes and thus these patients are in severe distress with low cardiac output and/or shock upon evaluation.

PRESENTATION

Acute decompensated AI causes pulmonary edema resulting in shortness of breath. The sudden regurgitant volume causes an increase in left-ventricular (LV) end-diastolic volume and left-atrial pressure. Because there is no time for the left ventricle to compensate for this increased volume, effective stroke volume acutely decreases. Tachycardia results to compensate but patients present with pulmonary edema and often shock despite having adequate blood pressure due to increased vascular resistance. Thus, these patients present with peripheral vasoconstriction, cyanosis, and appear gravely ill.

PHYSICAL EXAMINATION

- Diastolic murmur (blowing diastolic decrescendo murmur that may be soft or absent acutely).
- Tachycardia
- Pulmonary edema
- Look for Marfanoid characteristics

ACUTE MANAGEMENT

Diagnostic Tests:

- **CXR:** evaluate for signs of congestive heart failure; left-ventricle or left-atrial size are typically normal
- **TTE:** Evaluation for acute aortic insufficiency should include the following:
  - continuous wave Doppler to evaluate for a shortened pressure half time (<300 ms)
  - short mitral deceleration time (<150 ms)
  - premature closure of the mitral valve (may be assessed by M-mode)
  - reversed doming of the anterior mitral valve leaflet
  - evaluation of regurgitant jet width to LVOT diameter
  - suprasternal notch view to evaluate for flow reversal in the descending aorta and rule out aortic dissection
- **TEE:** May be considered for evaluation of the aortic valve for:
  - endocarditis or aortic valve ring abscess
  - rule out aortic dissection

Management:

- **Tools:** Swan-Ganz catheter for hemodynamic assessment, arterial line, IV access
- **STAT labs:** CBC, CMP, PT, INR, PTT, type and screen, blood cultures

Medications (depend on etiology):

- If acute aortic insufficiency is due to endocarditis or abscess, treat with antibiotics and IV afterload therapy
- If acute aortic insufficiency is due to a dissection, immediate surgery is indicated
- If acute aortic insufficiency is due to prosthetic valve leak or dehiscence, then treat with IV afterload therapy
- Consider rapid atrial or ventricular pacing if the patient is in cardiogenic shock

Surgical: Immediate surgical consultation is warranted especially in the setting of heart failure

CCU Tip: Temporary pacing may be necessary in severely decompensated patients to increase heart rate and cardiac output. Beta blockers in the setting of tachycardia with acute insufficiency can cause acute decompensation and cardiogenic shock and should be avoided.

- Widened pulse pressure—may not be present acutely
- Pulsus paradoxicus (seen with aortic dissection and pericardial effusion)
- Pulsus bisfierens

DIFFERENTIAL DIAGNOSIS

Leaflet Etiologies
- Endocarditis
- Leaflet Perforation
- Myxomatous valve
- Calcific aortic valve
- Rheumatic valve
- Congenital bicuspid, unicuspid, or quadricuspid valve
- Nonbacterial endocarditis (Libman-Sachs vegetations)
- Ventricular septal defect with prolapse of an aortic cusp
- Leaflet fenestration (due to amyloid, collagen vascular disorder, muco-polysaccharidosis, or glycogen storage disease)

Aortic Root Etiologies
- Aortic dissection*
- Dissecting ascending aortic aneurysm*
- Chest trauma*
- Marfan's syndrome*
- Cystic medial necrosis
- Hypertensive crisis with aortic root dilation*
- Systemic lupus erythematosus
- Ankylosing spondylitis

*More commonly present with acute AI.

- Giant cell aortitis
- Syphilitic aortitis
- Takayasu's aortitis
- Osteogenesis imperfecta

DIAGNOSTIC TESTS

Chest x-ray typically reveals a normal-sized LV and left-atrial (LA) in acute AI. Signs of congestive heart failure are very concerning in this setting.

Transthoracic echocardiography (TEE) may be indicated for AI that may be due to abnormalities of the aortic root or the leaflet themselves. Leaflet etiologies may be secondary due to changes in their flexibility or shape causing poor tip coaptation. Endocarditis can also cause regurgitation due to leaflet perforation or because a vegetation inhibits leaflet closure or creation of a perivalvular leak. Additionally, the mitral valve should be imaged as acute insufficiency can cause delayed opening of the valve and premature closure. The anterior leaflet of the mitral valve often has high-frequency fluttering but may not always be present in a calcified or rigid valve. Signs of severe AI include

- Regurgitant jet width to left ventricular outflow tract (LVOT) width ratio >60%
- Aortic regurgitant jet pressure half-time <300 ms

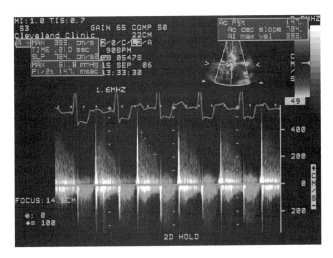

FIGURE 8.1. Pressure half-time <300 ms indicating severe AI.

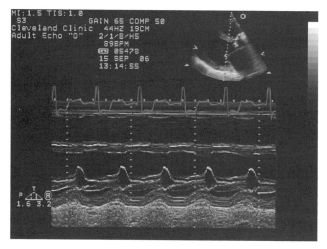

FIGURE 8.2. M-mode revealing premature closure of anterior mitral valve leaflet.

- Effective regurgitant orifice >0.30 cm^2
- Diastolic flow reversal in the descending aorta
- Reversed doming of the anterior mitral valve leaflet
- Premature closure of the mitral valve

TEE is useful in identifying suspected endocarditis, leaflet perforation, or an aortic root abscess. Additionally, TEE may be preferred in

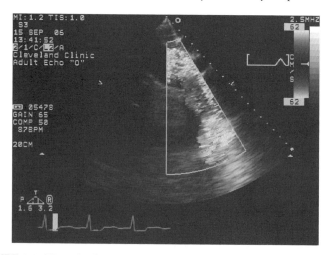

FIGURE 8.3. Diastolic flow reversal in the descending aorta.

evaluating prosthetic valve endocarditis or paravalvular leak and may be useful in identifying a bicuspid valve. Finally, the aorta can be evaluated for an ascending dissection with the same sensitivity as MRI or CT.

MEDICAL MANAGEMENT

Initial assessment should be made to determine the potential etiology of the insufficiency and the clinical state of the patient.

- Check for signs of blunt trauma.
- Check for marfanoid characteristics.
- Check the patients extremities for Osler nodes, Janeway lesions, Roth spots, and peripheral emboli suggestive of endocarditis.
- Palpate the patients chest for possible LV heave suggestive of LV overload.
- Evaluate for a bifid pulse.
- Determine pulse rate and pulse pressure.
- Determination of the etiology of AI is critical to management.

If the AI is due to aortic dissection and is severe then immediate surgery is required. Pain control should be used; judicious use of beta blockers can be considered. However, if the etiology of insufficiency is not due to dissection, then extreme care must be utilized with beta blockers as the tachycardia is compensatory. Beta blockade in this situation may precipitate cardiogenic shock, and worsen the patient's clinical status.

If the AI is due to endocarditis, vasodilator therapy with sodium nitroprusside can help reduce afterload if the patient has blood pressure to tolerate this therapy. Antibiotics should be started expeditiously after blood cultures have been drawn and chosen depending on the suspected pathogen.

In the setting of severe hypotension, an inotrope may be necessary for hemodynamic support. In this setting, norepinephrine may worsen the AI by increasing afterload and dopamine or dobutamine, either of which will increase heart rate, should be considered.

If the etiology is not due to dissection, then rapid atrial or ventricular pacing may improve the cardiac output by decreasing the diastolic filling time.

SURGICAL MANAGEMENT

Patients with severe acute AI should be seen immediately by a surgical consult team. In the setting of a Stanford Type A (Debakey types I or II) dissection, the patient should proceed directly to the operating room. Even in the setting of endocarditis, patients may necessitate emergent surgical replacement of the aortic valve depending on their hemodynamic status.

CLINICAL PRESENTATION TIPS

- Tachycardia is a compensatory response, which increases cardiac output in this setting. Beta blockers should not be utilized unless aortic dissection is a factor, and then only judiciously.
- Bradycardia may suggest aortic dissection progressing down the right coronary artery or endocarditis with an aortic ring abscess.
- Conduction abnormalities can be indicative of aortic ring abscess.
- Respiratory distress indicates acute worsening heart failure. Patients may need diuresis and consideration of a Swan-Ganz catheter to optimize their fluid status, and monitor afterload therapy in the setting of hypotension.
- Mental-status changes may suggest embolic phenomenon from the aortic valve or low cardiac output.
- Decreased urine output may also suggest embolic phenomena to the kidneys or low cardiac output.

DISCHARGE

Patients with acute severe AI should not be discharged from the intensive care unit (ICU) until a definitive diagnosis of etiology is made and the patient is stabilized hemodynamically. Often, patients with acute decompensated AI will not leave the ICU until proceeding to surgery.

RECOMMENDED READING

1. Bonow RO, et al. ACC/AHA 2006 guidelines for the management of patients with valvular heart disease: a report of the American College of Cardiology/American Heart Association Task Force on Practice Guidelines. *Circulation.* 2006; 114:84–231.
2. Otto C. Valvular regurgitation: diagnosis, quantitation, and clinical approach. In: Otto CM, ed. *Textbook of Clinical Echocardiography.* 2nd ed. Philadelphia: WB Saunders; 2000:277–285.

CHAPTER 9

Mitral Stenosis

APUR KAMDAR

Mitral stenosis (MS) is predominately caused by rheumatic heart disease and typically follows a slow progression over 10 to 20 years in the United States and Western Europe. Untreated, symptomatic patients have a 5-year mortality rate between 45% to 60%. Acute progression of this usually chronic condition requires prompt diagnosis, intensive care unit (ICU) admission, and treatment. Other causes include functional MS due to mobile masses in the left atrium including myxomas.

PRESENTATION

Critical MS, defined as mitral-valve opening ≤ 1 cm^2, results in an elevation of mean left-atrial (LA) pressure and pulmonary-venous pressures, usually manifesting as progressive exertional dyspnea, shortness of breath, and higher risk of developing atrial fibrillation and pulmonary hypertension. An elevated heart rate may exacerbate these symptoms by shortening diastolic flow time across the mitral valve and can result in sudden frank pulmonary edema in a previously asymptomatic patient.

PHYSICAL EXAMINATION

- Low-pitched, rumbling diastolic murmur at apex
- Diminished S$_1$ indicates advanced mitral disease
- Opening snap after S$_2$
- Accentuated P$_2$ suggesting pulmonary hypertension
- Diastolic thrill at apex in left lateral decubitus position

ACUTE MANAGEMENT

Diagnostic Tests:

- **ECG:** Not sensitive for mitral stenosis, but often has the following characteristics:
  - left-atrial enlargement
  - right-ventricular hypertrophy
  - atrial fibrillation
- **CXR:** Evaluate for signs of congestive heart failure
  - left-atrial enlargement may be seen
  - right-ventricular enlargement
  - mitral-valvular calcification may be appreciated
- **TTE:** Evaluation for severe mitral stenosis should include the following:
  - characteristic doming of the anterior mitral valve leaflet (hockey stick shaped) leaflet tip calcification (as opposed to leaflet base calcification) (Fig. 9.1)
  - poor leaflet separation in diastole
  - mitral-valve area by planimetry in short axis
  - left-atrial enlargement
  - Doppler hemodynamics revealing an elevated mean gradient
  - elevated pulmonary pressures
  - suitability for percutaneous balloon valvuloplasty if necessary
- **TEE:** Should be utilized to
  - rule out left-atrial and left-atrial appendage thrombus prior to percutaneous mitral valvuloplasty
  - evaluate mitral-valve morphology and hemodynamics when TTE is inadequate
  - prepare for potential percutaneous balloon valvuloplasty

Management:

- **Tools:** Swan-Ganz catheter for hemodynamic assessment, arterial line, IV access, nasal cannulae oxygen, foley catheter
- **STAT labs:** CBC, CMP, PT, INR, PTT, type and screen,

Medications:

- Beta-blocker therapy should be implemented for rate control
- Antiarrhythmic therapy (i.e., amiodarone) should be considered if new atrial fibrillation

- Diuretics to improve volume status and decrease congestion
- Salt-restricted diet
- Anticoagulation with heparin to prevent thromboembolic disease especially with atrial fibrillation or if thromboembolic event suspected
- Cardioversion should be considered for atrial fibrillation and hemo-dynamic collapse (rule out left atrial appendage thrombus first by transesophageal echocardiography)

Surgical: Consider percutaneous balloon mitral valvuloplasty if the valve appears suitable (less calcified, less subvalvular involvement), if the patient is pregnant or has severe medical comorbidities. If there is 2+ mitral regurgitation, left-atrial/appendage thrombus, or subvalvular involvement then consider surgical evaluation for replacement with possible Maze procedure.

CCU Tip: Beta blockers may be used even in cardiogenic shock and may actually improve cardiac output as long as LV function is not severely reduced, tachycardia is not present, and there is evidence of severe mitral stenosis. If a Swan-Ganz catheter is utilized, remember that the wedge pressure is falsely elevated. Pulmonary pressures greater than 60 mmHg usually indicate the need for intervention (valvuloplasty or surgery) regardless of symptoms.

- Elevated neck veins
- Pulmonary congestion, wheezing
- Clinical signs of hypoperfusion or cardiogenic shock
- Reduced pulse pressure, indicative of decreased stroke volume
- Signs of right-heart failure and/or pulmonary hypertension
- Peripheral cyanosis

DIFFERENTIAL DIAGNOSIS

- Congenital membrane in the left atrium
- Pulmonary vein obstruction
- LA tumor, myxoma causing obstruction to LA outflow
- Left-ventricular (LV) diastolic dysfunction

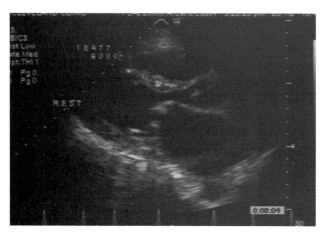

FIGURE 9.1. Severe mitral stenosis with diastolic doming and restricted leaflet motion. Note the classic hockey-stick appearance of the anterior leaflet.

- Cor triatriatum
- Mitral prosthetic valve thrombosis or degeneration

CAUSES AND RISK FACTORS

- Rheumatic fever (usual cause)
- Atrial fibrillation (rapid rate more than loss of atrial function critical in deterioration)
- Pregnancy (increased volume load and heart rate)
- Renal failure (increases calcification of valves and may cause stensosis)
- Carcinoid syndrome (rare)
- Congenital (rare, usually abnormal papillary muscle/chordal insertion)
- Systemic lupus erythematosus (rare, more usually mitral regurgitation [MR])
- Mucopolysaccharidoses diseases
- Infective endocarditis with large vegetations (rare)

DIAGNOSTIC TESTS

ECG

If the patient is in sinus rhythm, P-mitrale (Bifid P wave of increased duration) is indicative of LA enlargement

Chest X-Ray

Almost all patients with significant MS have LA enlargement that can be noted on CXR. This may be accompanied by enlarged pulmonary arteries and right-atrial (RA) and right-ventricular (RV) enlargement. Mitral-valvular calcification can also be noted and pulmonary congestion is an ominous finding.

TTE

- Mitral-valve area of less than 1.0 cm^2 by planimetry and pressure half time is indicative of severe mitral stenosis.

$$\text{Mitral-valve area} = 220/\text{pressure half time}$$

- Mean mitral-valve gradient $\geq$5 mmHg indicates some degree of MS; >10 mmHg usually indicates severe stenosis.
- Assess LA size.
- Assess LV function (often in chronic late disease).
- Pulmonary pressure $\geq$60 mmHg indicates the need for intervention regardless of symptoms.
- Planimetry of mitral valve.

Transesophageal Echo

Transesophageal echo (TEE) is useful if transthoracic echo cannot adequately determine the morphology or hemodynamics of the mitral valve. Additionally, if balloon valvuloplasty is considered or atrial fibrillation is a factor, TEE should be utilized to rule out LA or appendage thrombus.

Swan-Ganz Catheter

Generally, this technique should be avoided; however, it may be necessary when interpreting data with severe MS. As in all cases of low-output cardiac failure, the cardiac output by thermodilution is not accurate and should be calculated by the Fick method.

MEDICAL MANAGEMENT

Initial physical exam should include an assessment of volume status by examining jugular venous distension, pulmonary congestion, peripheral edema, and ascites. MS is associated with thromboembolic risk and signs of peripheral emboli should be noted. The cardiac rhythm, especially atrial fibrillation, should be noted given the association with decompensated heart failure in the setting of MS.

Intravenous access should be secured with basic laboratory studies including coagulation factors.

The goal in patients with low cardiac output due to MS is to identify the precipitating cause. In the intensive care unit (ICU), this commonly presents as an acute decompensated heart failure due to volume overload or secondary to atrial fibrillation. Therapy is directed to improve diastolic LV filling by decreasing the heart rate with intravenous metoprolol. Hemodynamically unstable patients with atrial fibrillation or any arrhythmias should be cardioverted and anticoagulated with unfractionated heparin. With severe hypotension, neosynephrine may provide a theoretical benefit due to its bradycardic effects. Diuresis as well as a low-sodium diet should also be considered.

Pregnancy can unmask occult MS by causing volume overload and acutely worsening heart failure. In this case, beta blockers and diuretics are once again beneficial and balloon valvuloplasty can be performed with excellent outcomes.

SURGICAL MANAGEMENT

Decompensated cardiac failure due to MS may be considered for percutaneous balloon valvuloplasty as well as an open surgical replacement of the mitral valve. Balloon valvuloplasty is considered the treatment of choice in appropriate patients with MS. A mitral-valve splittability score should be calculated to determine patients who will benefit most from this approach.

COMPLICATIONS

Cardiogenic shock may occur due to low cardiac output causing hypotension, severe fatigue, and acute renal failure with other end-organ sequelae.

Congestive heart failure occurs with the rise in LA pressure due to obstruction of flow across the mitral valve causing dyspnea, orthopnea, and paroxysmal nocturnal dyspnea. Tachycardia from any cause may exacerbate these symptoms by shortening diastolic flow time across the mitral valve. This can result in frank pulmonary edema in a previously asymptomatic patient within a short period of time.

Pulmonary hypertension occurs as LA pressure is transmitted to the pulmonary vasculature. Pulmonary pressures ≥ 60 mmHg indicates that an intervention should be made regardless of symptoms. Chronic pulmonary hypertension with RV dysfunction can manifest as liver dysfunction and ascites.

ECHO SCORE FOR VALVULOPLASTY

Calcification
1—single area of increased brightness
2—scattered areas of brightness located only on the leaflet margins
3—brightness extends to the mid portion of the leaflets
4—brightness extends throughout the leaflet tissue

Mobility
1—mobile mitral valve with restricted leaflet tips only
2—mild restriction of the leaflets with normal mobility at the base
3—valve moves forward in diastole mainly at the base
4—minimal movement of the leaflets in diastole

Thickening
1—normal leaflet thickness (4–5 mm)
2—thickened leaflets at the margins (5–8 mm)
3—thickened leaflets throughout the entire valve (5–8 mm)
4—severe thickening of the entire leaflet (8–10 mm)

Subvalvular apparatus
1—minimal thickening just below the leaflets
2—thickened chordae up to one third of the chordal length
3—thickened chordae to the distal third of the chordal length
4—extensive thickening and shortening of all chordal structures to the papillary muscles

CLINICAL PRESENTATION TIPS

a. Tachycardia is typically an atrial arrhythmia. Beta blockers and rhythm control are necessary.
b. Respiratory distress usually indicates heart failure and so diuretics must be implemented. Consideration should also be given for venous thromboembolic disease. Congested lungs in MS are more prone to infection so an accompanying respiratory infection should also be considered.
c. Decreased urine output may suggest either embolic phenomena or a low cardiac output state.
d. Mental-status changes may also suggest embolic event to the brain or low cardiac output.

Atrial fibrillation often occurs due to increased LA dilatation due to the stenotic mitral valve.

Thromboembolic disease is a concern in this population given the tendency of these patients to develop a LA or appendage thrombus.

DISCHARGE

Patients with severe MS requiring intensive care monitoring can be safely discharged from the intensive care unit (ICU) once their heart rate, rhythm, and hemodynamic status are stabilized. Beta-blocker therapy typically with metoprolol should be instituted and if necessary an anti-arrhythmic agent such as amiodarone should be used (assuming no liver dysfunction). Diuresis with furosemide and a sodium restricted diet will help optimize the patient's fluid status. Once these issues are addressed, the patient can be considered for percutaneous balloon valvuloplasty or surgical mitral-valve replacement.

RECOMMENDED READING

1. Bonow RO, et al. ACC/AHA 2006 guidelines for the management of patients with valvular heart disease: a report of the American College of Cardiology/American Heart Association Task Force on Practice Guidelines. *Circulation.* 2006; 114:84–231.
2. Otto C. Valvular stenosis: diagnosis, quantitation, and clinical approach. In: Otto CM, ed. *Textbook of Clinical Echocardiography.* 3rd ed. Philadelphia: WB Saunders; 2004.
3. Thamilarasan M, et al. Mitral valve disease. In: Griffen BP, Topol EJ, eds. *Manual of Cardiovascular Medicine.* 2nd ed. Philadelphia: Lippincott Williams & Wilkins; 2004:216–225.

CHAPTER 10

Mitral Regurgitation

DEEPU S. NAIR

The mitral valve (MV) is a complex structure composed of the mitral annulus, valve leaflets, chordae tendinae, papillary muscles, and underlying left-ventricular (LV) wall. Mitral regurgitation (MR) is caused by a variety of primary disorders of the valvular apparatus and also can be caused secondarily by processes altering LV geometry. Severe MR can be the result of progressive worsening of a degenerative valvular process, an acute mechanical complication of myocardial infarction (MI) (Chapter 2), or the result of endocarditis (Chapter 12).

The development of severe MR after acute MI often indicates papillary muscle dysfunction and can be rapidly fatal if not treated aggressively. In several studies, some degree of MR could be detected in up to 50% of patients after MI, with severe MR found in 12%. Understanding the underlying mechanism of MR can be vital for appropriate therapy.

In the setting of acute MR, a sudden volume overload is imposed on a nonhypertrophied, nondilated left atrium and left ventricle, resulting in pulmonary congestion and heart failure. Without medical and/or surgical therapy, the natural history of severe MR in the setting of acute myocardial infarction is progressive pulmonary congestion with low cardiac output that may lead to death. Patients with chronic MR can present with severe congestive heart failure (CHF) and require management similar to that employed in postinfarct MR.

PRESENTATION

The most common presentation of acute MR is new or worsening CHF, with findings including dyspnea, orthopnea, and lower-extremity edema. A history of recent acute MI or, rarely, chest trauma precedes

ACUTE MANAGEMENT

Diagnostic Tests:

- **ECG:** Possible findings include left-atrial enlargement, atrial fibrillation, LVH, or underlying myocardial infarction.
- **CXR:** Left-atrial enlargement, interstitial pulmonary edema
- **TTE:** Identify presence, severity, and mechanism of mitral regurgitation, specifically identifying presence of papillary muscle rupture, left-ventricle dysfunction, or vegetation. Color Doppler flow and continuous-wave Doppler studies can assess severity of regurgitation. Also, left-ventricle dimensions, size, and function of right ventricle, and pulmonary artery systolic pressure can be measured. It is not uncommon to have a TTE that does not reveal the true severity of mitral regurgitation.
- **TEE:** Higher resolution images of mitral-valve anatomy, allowing for precise characterization of mechanism and severity of mitral regurgitation. Consider when TTE images are suboptimal and prior to surgical intervention.

Management

- **Tools:**
  - Large bore IV line and/or central line, arterial line
  - Pulmonary artery catheter: in acutely decompensated patients
  - Intraortic balloon pump: in acutely decompensated patients with cardiogenic shock (e.g., papillary muscle rupture)
- Initial Labs: CBC, CMP, PT, INR, PTT

Medications:

- Afterload reduction
  - Nitroprusside gtt 0.1–8 µg/kg/min as needed up to 200 to 300 µg/min, titrating to improved hemodynamics (lower pulmonary capillary wedge pressure, higher SVO2)
  - Nitroglycerin gtt up to 200 µg/min—particularly with underlying ischemic disease
- Cardiac catheterization: In patients with suspected ischemic etiology or to assess coronary arteries prior to surgical intervention

Surgical evaluation

- Immediate surgical consultation with cardiothoracic surgery if acute severe mitral regurgitation

- General indications for surgery include symptomatic acute mitral regurgitation.

CCU Tips

- Patient presenting with postinfarct severe mitral regurgitation require immediate surgery and IABP insertion.
- Remember that a "normal" ejection fraction can represent left-ventricle dysfunction in the face of severe mitral regurgitation (EF should be above normal).
- Atrial fibrillation is a common complication of mitral regurgitation.
- Presence of pulmonary hypertension and/or right-ventricular dysfunction predicts worse outcome.
- TTE may underestimate mitral-regurgitation severity with eccentric jets.

papillary muscle rupture. Papillary muscle rupture often has a catastrophic presentation with frank cardiogenic shock manifested as hypotension and organ hypoperfusion. In contrast, chronic MR may be asymptomatic for years before presenting with symptoms of heart failure. In patients with underlying endocarditis, there can be a history of preceding febrile illness and evidence of systemic embolic phenomena. Rarely, features of Marfan's syndrome or other systemic connective-tissue disorders (e.g., Ehlers-Danlos syndrome) that can produce myxomatous MV degeneration will be found.

PHYSICAL EXAMINATION

- General: diaphoresis, change in mental status
- Neck: elevated jugular venous pressure (JVP), rapid descent of carotid pulse
- Cardiac: tachycardia, holosystolic "blowing" murmur at apex radiating to axilla (depends on direction of regurgitant jet and may be absent in acute MR), laterally displaced apical impulse (with LV dilatation), diminished S1 (in chronic MR), ±S3, ±RV heave and palpable P2 (if pulmonary hypertension has developed)
- Lungs: rales
- Extremities: peripheral edema (may not be present in acute setting), cold, clammy, mottled

DIFFERENTIAL DIAGNOSIS

Entities with Systolic Murmurs
- Ventricular septal defect (after MI)
- Tricuspid regurgitation
- Aortic stenosis
- Hypertrophic cardiomyopathy (LV outflow tract murmur)

RISK FACTORS

- Myxomatous MV disease
- Rheumatic heart disease
- Myocardial ischemia involving the papillary muscles
- Inferior MI may be more likely to cause papillary muscle rupture, as the posteromedial papillary muscle has a single blood supply (PDA), while the anterolateral papillary muscle has dual supply (LAD and LCx).
- LV dilatation
- Infectious endocarditis
- Congenital abnormalities (e.g., transposition of the great arteries, anomalous coronary artery)
- Connective tissue disorder (e.g., Marfan's syndrome, Ehlers-Danlos syndrome)
- Trauma
- Drugs (e.g., fenfluramine)

DIAGNOSTIC TESTS

Diagnostic imaging should be utilized to characterize the extent and underlying mechanism of MR, as well as to identify other coexisting structural lesions. Each part of the mitral-valve structure and perivalvular area, from the valve leaflets to supporting chordae and papillary muscles, should be carefully interrogated to identify redundancy, abnormal motion, or rupture. The chronicity of MR can be gauged by evaluating left-atrial size, pulmonary pressure, RV function and wall thickness. Transthoracic echocardiography (TTE) is generally the preferred initial study in patients with suspected mitral regurgitation.

TTE should be performed as soon as possible after the patient's arrival in the intensive care unit (ICU). A full study with careful attention to color Doppler flow and continuous wave Doppler flow across the

Etiologies of Mitral Regurgitation

Underlying Disease	Mechanism of Mitral Regurgitation
Myxomatous degeneration of mitral valve	Excess leaflet motion
Rheumatic heart disease	Restricted leaflet motion
Endocarditis	Destruction of valve tissue
Coronary artery disease	
– Papillary muscle rupture	Flail leaflet and papillary muscle
– Ischemia of posteromedial or adjacent left-ventricle wall	Abnormal chordal tethering
– Infarction of posteromedial or adjacent left ventricle wall	Chordal tethering, restricted motion
Dilated cardiomyopathy	Incomplete leaflet coaptation from altered posteromedial—annulus geometry

mitral valve should be performed once the patient has been stabilized. Left-atrial size, LV dimensions, pulmonary-artery-systolic pressure (via measurement of tricuspid regurgitant jet velocity), and LV systolic function should be assessed (Fig. 10.1). An assessment of MR severity can be made from echocardiographic features including size of the regurgitant jet by color Doppler, presence of proximal flow convergence, proximal isovelocity surface area (PISA), and extent of systolic pulmonary vein flow reversal. An early diastolic filling pulse-wave (E wave) velocity >1.2 m/sec may be suggestive of significant MR.

Transesophageal echocardiography (TEE) can provide excellent visualization of the mitral-valve anatomy and has higher sensitivity for pathologic entities associated with MR. TEE is particularly important in obese patients or those with poor transthoracic windows, patients with prosthetic valves, and patients for whom surgical repair is planned. In patients with suspected papillary muscle rupture, TEE should nearly always be performed as the regurgitant jet may be eccentric and difficult to detect by TTE.

Magnetic resonance imaging (MRI) can quantify regurgitant flow with high accuracy but its use is limited by long acquisition time.

Cardiac catheterization is now rarely used as a primary means of diagnosing MR. It can be useful therapeutically in patients with MR due to papillary muscle ischemia and is required to assess coronary anatomy prior to mitral-valve surgery.

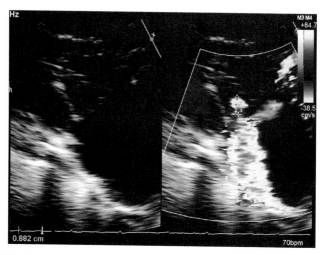

FIGURE 10.1. Parasternal long-axis view of the mitral valve in patient with mitral regurgitation. Left panel shows anterior MV leaflet prolapse. Right panel shows regurgitant jet, with crosses indicating radius of proximal flow convergence.

MEDICAL MANAGEMENT

On arrival to the ICU, initial attention should be focused on physical examination, including measurement of vital signs such as arm blood pressures, identification of jugular venous distention (JVD) and careful cardiac auscultation. Cardiac exam may reveal the classic holosystolic blowing murmur of MR with radiation to the axilla or base (depending on the direction of the regurgitant jet) as well as presence of S3. Pulmonary exam may reveal rales and pleural effusions depending on the acuity of the MR. The extremities should be inspected for edema and for peripheral stigmata of endocarditis (e.g., Janeway lesions, Osler's nodes).

Two large-bore intravenous (IV) sites and a radial arterial line should be placed for administration of vasoactive medications and close hemodynamic monitoring, respectively. Consideration should be given to the placement of a central venous catheter in unstable patients to allow rapid medication delivery.

A pulmonary artery catheter can be useful for management of patients with hemodynamic compromise and impaired oxygenation, as it may guide optimal titration of afterload reducing agents. It will also help determine whether pulmonary hypertension is present, and whether it is fixed or reversible.

The goal of medical therapy in acute MR is afterload reduction, which decreases systemic vascular resistance, improves forward cardiac output, and lessens regurgitant flow. If adequate systemic blood pressure is present, treatment with intravenous sodium nitroprusside should be initiated, beginning at a low dose (e.g., 0.5 to 1 µg/kg/min) and titrating upward as blood pressure allows. In our cardiac intensive care unit (CICU) such patients are frequently treated with doses as high as 200 to 300 µg/min. In general, the goal is to maintain a mean arterial pressure of 55 to 60 mmHg in patients without evidence of coronary artery disease (CAD) and a mean arterial pressure of 65 to 70 mmHg in those with CAD.

IV nitroglycerin can also be used as an effective venodilator, particularly in patients with an underlying ischemic etiology for MR. If used, nitroglycerin should be started at a low dose (e.g., 20 µg/min) and titrated upward with continuous hemodynamic monitoring.

Vasodilators cannot be used as first-line therapy in patients with hypotension in acute MR. These patients require acute hemodynamic support with an IABP. The IABP primarily reduces afterload, thereby improving cardiac performance in this setting.

Unlike in mitral stenosis (MS), heart-rate management is somewhat less critical in patients with MR, as regurgitant flow is primarily a systolic phenomenon and systolic ejection time varies less with changing heart rate.

PERCUTANEOUS MANAGEMENT

Reduction in MR has been reported after percutaneous intervention in patients with severe MR due to ischemia of the papillary muscle rather than frank rupture. However, direct surgical intervention is necessary in cases of papillary muscle rupture.

SURGICAL MANAGEMENT

Acute MR with hemodynamic compromise usually requires immediate surgical intervention, particularly in cases of papillary muscle rupture. Options for treatment include mitral-valve repair and mitral-valve replacement. Operative mortality for papillary muscle rupture can be 20% to 50%, but surgery should still be considered in every patient since medical therapy alone has higher mortality. Surgical treatment of ischemic MR often requires concomitant CABG. When possible, the surgeon will try to preserve the subvalvular apparatus to limit postoperative deterioration of LV function. MV repair is feasible in cases where the valve leaflets, chordae, and annulus are not too disrupted by the underlying disease process. Exceptions that may require MV replacement include extensive chordal rupture, endocarditis with valve destruction, and rheumatic heart disease with extensive annular calcification. In patients with MR in the setting of dilated cardiomyopathy, MV repair may result in symptomatic improvement but a survival benefit has not yet been shown. Whenever possible, surgical intervention should be pursued before left-ventricular ejection fraction (LVEF) drops to the subnormal (<60%) range as delay results in worse outcomes.

CLINICAL PRESENTATION TIPS

- Hypotension—suspect flail leaflet or papillary muscle rupture
- Preceding angina—consider papillary muscle ischemia and/or rupture
- Fever—suspect mitral-valve endocarditis with associated valve dysfunction or perforation
- Embolic phenomena—suspect mitral-valve endocarditis
- Palpitations—anticipate atrial fibrillation, as it is commonly seen with mitral regurgitation

COMPLICATIONS

CHF develops when severe MR results in decreased effective forward cardiac output, elevated pulmonary capillary wedge measure (PCWP) and pulmonary edema. CHF represents the most common mechanism of death in patients with acute MR. Evidence of pulmonary congestion and/or hypotension requires vasodilator therapy, IABP, and/or surgery as discussed previously.

Endocarditis can cause MR, but conversely, the abnormal structure and flow pattern around a dysfunctional valve can predispose to developing endocarditis.

Atrial fibrillation (AF) can be the result of acute left-atrial volume overload and stretch due to MR. Management may include rate control or direct current cardioversion if unstable. Occasionally, patients undergoing mitral-valve surgery will additionally undergo MAZE procedure to treat atrial fibrillation. The success of this procedure has been reported to range from 60% to 75%.

Post-MI mortality is markedly higher in patients who develop MR after an ischemic event. If associated with cardiogenic shock, the mortality rate could be as high as 50%.

DISCHARGE

The majority of patients with acute MR and hemodynamic compromise will require urgent surgery. Discharge from the ICU is possible in patients with less severe MR once pulmonary congestion has improved, blood pressure has normalized, and an adequate oral medication regimen has been instituted. Oral vasodilators including ACE-I or hydralazine and nitrates are the preferred medications. Beta blockers may be beneficial but should be started once adequate afterload reduction has been achieved. In patients with pulmonary congestions, nitrates and diuretics may also be needed. It should, however, be noted that vasodilator therapy can "mask" the severity of MR, potentially causing a delay in timing of surgery.

RECOMMENDED READING

1. Bursi F, et al. Mitral regurgitation after myocardial infarction: a review. *Am J Med.* 2006; 119(2):103–112.
2. Thompson CR, et al. Cardiogenic shock due to acute severe mitral regurgitation complicating acute myocardial infarction: a report from the SHOCK Trial Registry. Should we use emergently revascularize occluded coronaries in cardiogenic shock? *J Am Coll Cardiol.* 2000; 36(3 Suppl A):1104–1109.
3. Topol EJ. *Textbook of Cardiovascular Medicine.* 2nd ed. Philadelphia: Lippincott Williams & Wilkins; 2002:2210.
4. Iwasaki K, et al. Transesophageal echocardiography for detection of mitral regurgitation due to papillary muscle rupture or dysfunction associated with acute myocardial infarction: a report of five cases. *Can J Cardiol.* 2000; 16(10):1273–1277.
5. Dekker AL, et al. Intra-aortic balloon pumping in acute mitral regurgitation reduces aortic impedance and regurgitant fraction. *Shock.* 2003; 19(4): 334–338.
6. Pellizzon GG, et al. Importance of mitral regurgitation inpatients undergoing percutaneous coronary intervention for acute myocardial infarction: the controlled abciximab and device investigation to lower late angioplasty complications (CADILLAC) trial. *J Am Coll Cardiol.* 2004; 43(8):1368–1374.

7. Pierard LA, Lancellotti P. The role of ischemic mitral regurgitation in the pathogenesis of acute pulmonary edema. *N Engl J Med.* 2004; 351(16): 1627–1634.
8. Lamas GA. Clinical significance of mitral regurgitation after acute myocardial infarction. Survival and ventricular enlargement investigators. *Circulation.* 1997; 96(3):827–833.
9. Grayburn PA. Vasodilator therapy for chronic aortic and mitral regurgitation. *Am J Med Sci.* 2000; 320(3): 202–208.

CHAPTER 11

Tricuspid Valvular Disease

MATHEW C. BECKER

ricuspid regurgitation (TR) is very common and can be observed in as many as 70% of "normal" patients. The etiology of TR can be divided into two categories depending on the etiology of valvular pathology. *Organic tricuspid disease* results from insults to the valvular components including the leaflets, annulus, or chordae. *Functional tricuspid disease* is a consequence of right-ventricular (RV) dilatation or elevation in left-sided pressures. The most common cause of TR is functional due to volume or pressure overload of the right ventricle.

PRESENTATION

While mild TR is common and generally well tolerated, greater degrees of insufficiency may result in a decrease in cardiac output and lead to significant symptoms. Fatigue, nuchal pulsation due to elevations in jugular venous pressure (JVP), right upper-quadrant abdominal pain, as well as massive peripheral edema may all be presenting complaints in the patient with moderate to severe TR.

PHYSICAL EXAMINATION

- General cachexia, weight loss, and jaundice
- Pulsatile jugular venous distention (JVD) and a prominent v wave peaking at S_2 with a sharp y descent
- Pansystolic murmur best auscultated at the left, lower sternal border. This may be accentuated with deep inspiration (Rivero-Carvallo

sign), abdominal pressure, inhalation of amyl nitrate or decreased with the Valsalva maneuver, standing position, or progressive RV failure
- Right-sided S_3 or S_4
- Early diastolic rumble that may be heard due to increased diastolic flow across the TV
- Enlarged, tender, and pulsatile liver
- Abdominal distention, fluid wave, and shifting dullness due to ascites
- Lower-extremity edema or anasarca in more severe disease

DIFFERENTIAL DIAGNOSIS

Functional Etiologies
- Pulmonary hypertension (from any cause, i.e., pulmonary embolism [PE], chronic obstructive pulmonary disease [COPD], cor pulmonale, pulmonic stenosis)
- Mitral stenosis (MS)
- Left-to-right shunt
- Left-sided CHF
- Hyperthyroidism

Organic Etiologies
- Myxomatous degeneration or rheumatic disease
- Ruptured chordae or papillary muscle
- Device-related injury (Swan-Ganz catheter or pacemaker wire)
- Drug related (Fen fen or Methysergide)
- Endocarditis
- Ebstein's anomaly, Fabry's or Whipple's disease

DIAGNOSTIC TESTS

ECG findings may be nonspecific but RV strain may be suggestive of tricuspid valve insufficiency. There may be nonspecific ST-T waves or

---

ACUTE MANAGEMENT

Diagnostic Tests:

- **ECG:** look for signs of right-ventricular strain such as right ventricular hypertrophy (RVH), right-axis deviation or right-atrial hypertrophy as evidenced by a "p pulmonale" in lead II. Also an S in lead I, Q in lead III and T-wave inversion in lead III can be suggestive of a pulmonary embolus.

- **CXR:** evaluate for signs of congestive heart failure and right-atrial or right-ventricle enlargement
- **TTE:** Evaluation for acute aortic insufficiency should include the following:
  - quantifying the severity of tricuspid regurgitation
  - calculating the RVSP using the modified Bernoulli equation (Pressure $= RAP + 4v^2$)
  - evaluating for right-atrial enlargement (area >20 cm^2)
  - evaluating right-ventricle size and function
  - checking for volume or pressure overload by assessing septal flattening
- **TEE:** typically is not considered as effective as TTE for the tricuspid valve but may be utilized to evaluate an organic cause of tricuspid regurgitation

Management:

- **Tools:** Swan-Ganz catheter for hemodynamic assessment, arterial line, IV access
- **STAT labs:** CBC, CMP, PT, INR, PTT, type and screen, blood cultures
- search for the underlying cause of the tricuspid regurgitation with

Medications (depend on the etiology):

- If acute tricuspid regurgitation is due to endocarditis, treat with antibiotics
- If acute tricuspid regurgitation is due to left ventricular failure, consider IV afterload therapy with nitroprusside ± nitroglycerin
- Diurese with furosemide in the setting of volume overload
- Anticoagulate with heparin if PE is a concern

Surgical: Surgery is typically not indicated in isolated tricuspid valve disease and valve repair must be considered in conjunction with the patient's comorbidities.

CCU Tip: The presence of an occult shunt such as an ASD or PFO is an important cause of idiopathic RV pressure or volume overload and should be sought by a TTE with an agitated saline study.

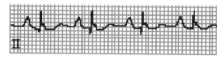

FIGURE 11.1. Right-atrial enlargement in setting of severe TR.

more commonly right-ventricular hyperthropy (RVH) with right-axis deviation or a right bundle branch block (RBBB). Additionally, the classic sign for a pulmonary embolus with an S in V6, Q in lead III and T-wave inversion in lead II may be seen. Finally, a "p-pulmonale" may suggest right-atrial strain due to severe tricuspid regurgitation (Fig. 11.1).

Chest x-ray findings typically reveal enlargement of the right atrium (RA) or RV and potentially signs of congestive heart failure (CHF) (Kerley-B lines, pulmonary edema, etc.).

Transthoracic echocardiography (TTE) shows the parasternal short axis, apical four-chamber, and subcostal views that provide optimal visualization of the tricuspid valve. Severe, functional TR will typically be accompanied by evidence of RV pressure or volume overload (Fig 11.2). An interatrial shunt (i.e., ASD or PFO) may cause an idiopathic increase in RV pressures and should be ruled out by subcostal Doppler imaging of the interatrial septum as well as by an agitated saline study.

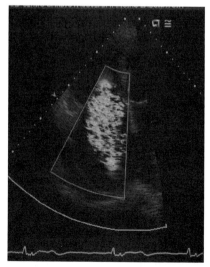

FIGURE 11.2. Color Doppler of severe TR in the apical four-chamber view.

The right ventricular systolic pressure (RVSP) can be calculated with the modified Bernoulli when an adequate continuous wave Doppler tracing is recorded across the TV. The right-trial pressure (RAP) should be added to this figure and can be approximated by either the size of the inferior vena cava (IVC) as it joins the RA ($<1.5 \sim 5$ mmHg; 1.5–$2.5 \sim 10$ mmHg; >2.5 cm ~ 15 mmHg). Thus, the RVSP = $RAP + 4v^2$.

Typical TTE findings of pressure overload include

- Right-atrial enlargement (RAE) (area >20 cm^2)
- RV dilatation ($>2/3$ the LV dimension) with systolic dysfunction
- Septal flattening (diastolic—more commonly associated with volume overload; systolic—more commonly associated with pressure overload)
- Systolic-flow reversal in the inferior vena cava (IVC) or hepatic veins—consistent with severe TR
- Dilatation of the IVC (>2.5 cm) or hepatic veins (0.5–1.0 cm)

TEE can be helpful in determining the etiology of tricuspid dysfunction or to inspect for vegetations when TTE imaging is insufficient. However, the TV and PV are more difficult to image with TEE than the mitral or aortic valves, because they are thinner and deeper into the far field requiring lower frequencies to adequately penetrate.

Right-heart catheterization uses a pulmonary artery catheter (PAC) or Swan-Ganz catheter to effectively evaluate pulmonary arterial hypertension. In addition, the PAC also allows for ongoing hemodynamic management of pulmonary arterial hypertension (PAH) with vasoactive therapies as discussed elsewhere in this text. Significant findings include

- venous pressure tracing with large V waves in significant TR
- severe TR may result in a significant *underestimation* of cardiac output when employing the thermodilutional method due to "washout" phenomenon
- in this setting, consider strictly using the Fick-derived cardiac output

MEDICAL MANAGEMENT

Initial management of the patient with severe tricuspid regurgitation should focus on determining the etiology. The physical exam should be suggestive of a potential cause. Tachypnea, tachycardia, RV heave, and decreased oxygen saturation is suggestive of a functional etiology (i.e., pulmonary hypertension from a PE or COPD, or left-sided heart failure). A diastolic murmur can be suggestive of MS. A fever, embolic phenomena, or drug use would be suggestive of organic valve disease from endocarditis or drug-related valvular damage.

If a PE is the cause, then heparin should be instituted and thrombolytic therapy given if cardiogenic shock develops.

In the setting of LV failure, sodium nitroprusside may be started for afterload reduction. If the LV failure has a component of unrevascularized myocardium, then nitroglycerin should be started first to prevent a coronary steal phenomenon. Additionally, diuretics may be considered in the setting of volume overload.

If endocarditis is the etiology of valve dysfunction, immediate antibiotic therapy should be incorporated (Chapter 12).

Surgical Evaluation

Patients with isolated tricuspid regurgitation typically do not need surgical repair. Any surgical intervention on the tricuspid valve should be considered in conjunction with the patient's other valvular or coronary comorbidities.

CLINICAL PRESENTATION AND COMPLICATIONS

- **Hypotension:** suspect left-ventricle dysfunction causing the tricuspid regurgiation

- **Respiratory distress:** acute heart failure from left-ventricle dysfunction, pulmonary embolism, and chronic obstructive pulmonary disease should be considered

---

DISCHARGE

Patients may be discharged from the coronary care unit (CCU) once they have been hemodynamically stabilized and the etiology for the tricuspid regurgitation is clearly defined and therapeutically addressed.

RECOMMENDED READING

1. Cheitlin MD, Macgregor JS. Acquired tricuspid and pulmonary valve disease. In: Topol et al. ed. *Textbook of Cardiovascular Medicine.* 2nd ed. Philadelphia: Lippincott-Raven Publishers; 2002:529–548.
2. Weyman AE. *Principles and Practice of Echocardiography.* 2nd ed. Philadelphia: Lea & Febiger; 1994: 824–862.

CHAPTER 12

Infective Endocarditis

BRET A. ROGERS

Infective endocarditis results in a wide array of clinical syndromes, ranging from subtle, subacute, febrile illness to acute cardiogenic shock with multisystem organ failure to subarrachnoid hemorrhage with changes in mental status. Care for patients with more severe cases of infective endocarditis should focus on timely and accurate assessment of affected cardiac structures, early appropriate antibiotic therapy, supportive care of associated complications, and referral for surgical intervention when this is necessary.

PRESENTATION

Patients presenting with infective endocarditis typically report symptoms including fever, malaise, fatigue, and weight loss, usually of 2 weeks' duration or less. Those patients requiring intensive care unit (ICU) admission typically have progressed to congestive heart failure (CHF) from valvular regurgitation, leaflet dysfunction, rupture perivalvular abscesses leading to fistula formation, or conduction abnormalities due to aortic ring abscess causing atrioventricular nodal dysfunction. Additionally, septic emboli may cause acute shortness of breath, chest pain, mental-status changes or renal failure.

PHYSICAL EXAMINATION

Features of the physical examination suggestive of infective endocarditis include

- Fever, tachycardia, tachypnea, hypotension (from septic or cardiogenic shock)

ACUTE MANAGEMENT

Diagnostic Tests:

- **ECG:** evaluates for signs of conduction disturbances
- **CXR:** is useful for evaluating acute congestive heart failure
- **TTE:** examines for vegetations on valves in multiple views, assess valve function and left ventricular function
- **TEE:** should be performed if endocarditis is considered and the TTE is nondiagnostic. Additionally, it should be performed if a perforated leaflet, ruptured chordae, abscess, or fistula is suspected or if there is intracardiac hardware (prosthesis, pacemaker wires) present.
- **CT/MRI:** may need to be performed if the patient has mental status changes as septic emboli to the brain may preclude a surgical intervention. Also may assess for mycotic aneurysm prior to surgical intervention.
- **Cerebral angiogram:** May be necessary to evaluate patients with mycotic aneurysm.

Management:

- **Tools:** IV access for antibiotics, ECG, portable CXR
- **STAT labs:** Blood cultures, CBC, CMP, PT/PTT, Type and Screen
- **Medications**
  - start empiric antibiotics immediately after blood cultures are drawn
  - an inotrope such as norepinephrine may be necessary in acute hypotension
  - consider diuresis with furosemide if significant congestion is present
  - if a conduction abnormality manifests, consider temporary venous pacing and suspect abscess formation (TEE may be needed to exclude)

Surgical: Emergent surgical evaluation is indicated in cases of severe aortic or mitral insufficiency, abscess or fistula formation, fungal infection, extremely large vegetations, or recurrent embolic phenomena.

> **CCU Tip:**
> - Have a low threshold to consider TEE.
> - Consider septic emboli if ECG changes (emboli to coronary artery usually with aortic valve IE) or patient becomes hemodynamically unstable, if urine output decreases, abdominal pain (ischemic bowel), mental-status change
> - Serial ECG to monitor abscess extension into conduction system

- Elevated jugular venous pressure (JVP)
- Bibasilar crackles
- New/changing heart murmurs
- Abdominal, visceral, or flank tenderness (from embolic phenomena)
- Splinter hemorrhages, Janeway lesions/Osler nodes, Roth spots
- Focal neurologic deficits
- Meningeal signs

DIFFERENTIAL DIAGNOSIS

- Noninfective endocarditis (marantic or Libman-Sachs)
- Thrombosis
- Intracardiac tumor
- Lambl's excrescence (strand-like structures seen in older patients)

RISK FACTORS

- Dental procedure, poor dental hygiene
- Intravenous drug abuse
- Hemodialysis patient or chronic indwelling venous catheter
- Endoscopic gastrointestinal or genitourinary procedure
- Immunocompromised state
- Chronic intracardiac devices including valves, pacemaker leads, and dialysis catheters

COMMON ORGANISMS

- Streptococci (viridans and bovis)
- Enterococci

- Staphylococci (both coagulase positive and negative)
- Gram negative aerobes
- Fungi
- HACEK (*Haemophilus, Actinobacillus, Cardiobacterium, Eikenella, Kingella*)

DIAGNOSTIC TESTS

Blood cultures are essential in establishing the diagnosis of endocarditis. Other relevant laboratory findings include an elevated white blood cell count, erythrocyte sedimentation rate, and rheumatoid factor. See the following Duke Criteria.

Electrocardiograms (ECG) may reveal a conduction disturbance, which is concerning for abscess formation. First-degree atrioventricular block in this setting is particularly concerning and should not be overlooked.

Transthoracic echocardiography (TTE) is the primary modality for diagnosing infective endocarditis in the acutely decompensated patient. Congenital heart abnormalities such as a bicuspid aortic valve should be ruled out.

Transesophageal echocardiography (TEE) is indicated when TTE does not adequately characterize the vegetation or mechanism of valvular dysfunction. It is especially useful when abscess or fistula formation is suspected (as in the case of conduction abnormalities) or when a perforated leaflet or ruptured chordae is suspected. Additionally, it should be utilized when there are intracardiac devices such as pacing wires and prosthetic valves due to its greater diagnostic yield.

CT/MRI of the brain may be necessary in cases in which patients present with acute mental-status changes or mental obtundation. Septic emboli to the brain may preclude surgical intervention of severe valvular disease. If the patient does have neurological deficits, a neurology consult will be necessary as these patients are at increased risk of bleeding if mycotic aneurysms are present.

MEDICAL MANAGEMENT

Initial management should include cardiac auscultation to evaluate for murmurs. Additionally, a brief focused exam for heart failure and signs of peripheral emboli should be conducted. Finally, a baseline neurological assessment should be performed. If there is a chronic indwelling catheter, pacemaker, or ICD in place, the site should be checked for tenderness, erythema, or pus.

DEFINITIONS FOR THE DUKE CRITERIA FOR THE DIAGNOSIS OF INFECTIVE ENDOCARDITIS

Clinical Criteria: Twp major, one major and three minor, or five minor criteria
Pathologic Criteria vegetation or abscess confirmed by histology

Major Criteria

- Positive Blood Culture:
  - typical microorganism from two separate cultures, or
  - persistently positive blood cultures drawn ≥12 hrs apart or from 3 of 4 cultures ≥1 hr apart

- Endocardial Involvement:
  - Positive echocardiogram for vegetation
    - Intracardiac mass on the valve or supporting structure
    - Abscess
    - New partial dehiscence of prosthetic valve
  - New valvular regurgitation

Minor Criteria

- Predisposing condition or behavior
- Fever ≥38.0° C
- Vascular phenomena: Septic infarcts or emboli, mycotic aneurysms, intracranial hemorrhage, Janeway lesions, conjunctival hemorrhages
- Immunologic phenomena: Roth spots, Osler nodes, Rheumatoid Factor, Glomerulonephritis
- Microbiologic evidence:
  - Positive blood culture not meeting major criteria
  - Serologic evidence of infection with typical organism of endocarditis
- Echo consistent with endocarditis not meeting the major criteria

Intravenous access should be rapidly obtained with blood cultures, complete blood count (CBC), erythrocyte sedimentation rate, and electrolytes. Baseline ECG and CXR should also be readily performed.

Broad-spectrum antimicrobial therapy should be implemented as soon as blood cultures are drawn pending speciation of the pathogen. Bactericidal therapy with penicillin-related antibiotics is most efficacious, but if there is a question of resistant pathogens, vancomycin should be utilized. An aminoglycoside has a synergistic effect during bacteremia and should be implemented carefully with consideration of renal function. Rifampin may be needed in the setting of prosthetic valve infection.

SURGICAL MANAGMENT

The likely source of the endocardial infection should be treated and/or removed prior to undergoing any surgical treatment. However, there are several emergent indications for surgery in this population. These include acute aortic insufficiency or mitral regurgitation with severe hemodynamic instability and heart failure. Abscess formation indicates the need for emergent surgery as does a fungal etiology. Other factors that may cause consideration for urgent operation include large (>10 mm) (greater risk of embolization) and recurrent embolic phenomena despite adequate antimicrobial therapy (Fig. 12.1). Endocarditis of mechanical prosthesis is not cured by antibiotic treatment alone and is an indication for surgical removal of the prosthesis and implantation of a homograft if this is feasible. Failure of appropriate antimicrobial treatment to eradicate the infection is another indication for surgery.

If cerebral embolization has occurred, preoperative cerebral angiography is indicated to assess for mycotic aneurysm formation; many experts believe that surgery should be delayed in this situation for 2 to 4 weeks following treatment of the aneurysm to reduce the risk of intracranial

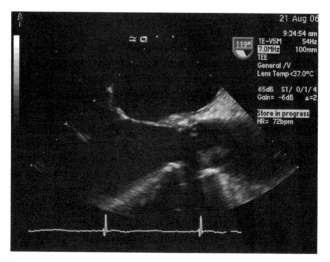

FIGURE 12.1. Bioprosthetic aortic valve abscess with vegetation (white arrow) and root abscess.

bleed during surgery, though surgery may be performed as early as 7 days if there are compelling clinical indications such as recurring embolization or worsening heart failure.

CLINICAL PRESENTATION TIPS

- Acute MI: may occur due to septic emboli via a coronary artery (most common with aortic valve endocarditis).
- Heart Block: likely due to abscess or fistula formation
- Mental status change: cerebral emboli or subarachnoid hemorrhage
- Respiratory Distress: due to acute heart failure from severe aortic or mitral insufficiency
- Renal Failure: emboli to the kidneys or antibiotic toxicity

---

COMPLICATIONS

CHF is generally caused by valvular dysfunction with regurgitant lesions resulting from leaflet perforation or disruption of normal coaptation. Functional obstruction can also result from bulky vegetations that partially occlude the affected valve orifice. Without surgical intervention, mortality is extremely high in patients developing this complication.

Conduction disturbances are usually caused by extension of an annular abscess into the conduction system. Patients with this complication may require temporary transvenous pacing until surgery, after which permanent pacing will likely be required.

Embolization is the most common extracardiac complication of endocarditis. While cerebral embolization and subsequent infarction/ hemorrhage are the most feared embolic phenomena, virtually all organ systems may be affected including the kidneys, spleen, gut, or limbs, and metastatic infections requiring surgical or percutaneous drainage. Right-sided endocarditis may be associated with septic pulmonary emboli, resulting in hemoptysis, pleural effusions, empyema, and/or pneumothorax.

DISCHARGE

In patients admitted to the ICU with endocarditis, discharge is usually contingent upon resolution of bacteremia and any associated complications. Most often, this occurs after surgical treatment of the infection, as it is CHF or conduction abnormalities that necessitate ICU care. Those patients admitted to ICUs for monitoring after embolic events (e.g., stroke) may be transferred to a step-down or intermediate care unit once stable.

RECOMMENDED READING

1. Bonow RV, Carabello B, de Leon AC, et al. Guidelines for the management of patients with valvular heart disease: executive summary: a report of the American College of Cardiology/American Heart Association Task Force of Practice Guidelines (Committee on Management of Patients with Valvular Heart Disease). *Circulation.* 1998; 98;1949–1984.
2. Durack DT, Lukes AS, Bright DK. New criteria for diagnosis of infective endocarditis: utilization of specific echocardiographic findings. Duke Endocarditis Service. *Am J Med.* 1994; 96:200–209.
3. Sexton DJ, Bashore TM. Infective endocarditis. In: Topol EJ, ed. *Textbook of Cardiovascular Medicine.* 2nd ed. Philadelphia: Lippincott Williams & Wilkins; 2002:569–593.
4. Wilson WR, Karchmer AW, Dajani AS, et al. Antibiotic treatment of adults with infective endocarditis due to streptococci, enterococci, staphylococci, and HACEK microorganisms. *JAMA.* 1995: 274:1706–1713.
5. Wallace SM, et al. Mortality from infective endocarditis: clinical predictors of outcome. *Heart.* 2002; 88:53–60.

CHAPTER 13

Prosthetic Valve Disease

YULI Y. KIM

Approximately 95,000 valve procedures were performed in the United States in 2003. Prosthetic heart valves are either mechanical or bioprosthetic. Mechanical valves range from *caged-ball* valves (Starr-Edwards), *single-tilting-disk* (Bjork-Shiley, Medtronic-Hall), and *bileaflet-tilting-disk* (St. Jude Medical, Carbomedics) models (Fig. 13.1). Bioprosthetic valves can be *heterografts* composed of porcine or bovine tissue typically mounted on a stent to which the leaflets and sewing ring are attached (Hancock, Carpentier-Edwards) (Fig. 13.2), *homografts* which are preserved human aortic valves, or pulmonary *autografts* in which the patient's own pulmonary valve is placed in the aortic position; the pulmonary valve is then replaced with a homograft or heterograft.

Prosthetic valves differ in terms of durability, thrombogenicity, and hemodynamic profile. Although mechanical valves afford a highly durable option, they are thrombogenic and require anticoagulation. On the other hand, bioprosthetic valves appear to be less thrombogenic but their durability is significantly less than that of mechanical valves (30% of heterografts and 10% to 20% of homografts require replacement within 10 to 15 years).

Complications of prosthetic valves that are encountered in the intensive care unit (ICU) setting include valve obstruction, thromboembolism, structural failure, endocarditis, paravalvular leak, hemolysis, and bleeding. All except the last are discussed next.

VALVE OBSTRUCTION

Background

Prosthetic valve obstruction may be caused by thrombus, pannus, degeneration, or vegetation. The estimated incidence of prosthetic valve

ACUTE MANAGEMENT

Diagnostic Tests:

- **CXR:** Evaluate for signs of congestive heart failure; dilated left ventricle or left atrium
- **TTE:** Should evaluate
  - disk movement
  - transvalvular gradient
  - presence of thrombus
  - valvular or paravalvular regurgitation
  - dimensionless index
- **TEE:** Is frequently necessary for suspected prosthetic valve dysfunction:
  - in addition to above features that are evaluated with TTE
  - close surveillance of thrombus size and leaflet/disk mobility
  - distinguish thrombus from pannus (thrombus tends to be more mobile)

Cinefluoroscopy:

- To assess disk motion and opening and closing angles

Management:

- **Tools:** May need pulmonary artery catheter for hemodynamic assessment
- Arterial line, IV access
- **STAT labs:** CBC, CMP, PT, INR, PTT, type and screen, blood cultures

Medications (depend on etiology):

- If valve obstruction is due to pannus formation, treatment is surgical replacement.
- If the thrombus is nonobstructive and <5 mm, it is often possible to treat with heparin alone while monitoring thrombus size with TEE.
- If obstructive thrombus, treatment strategies are valve replacement and/or thrombolysis; however, replacement is favored over thrombolysis due to a lower rate of recurrence.
- If right-sided valve thrombosis and patient is hemodynamically unstable then consider alteplase (10 mg bolus, then 90 mg over 90 minutes), streptokinase (500,000 IU over 20 minutes, then 1.5 MIU over 10 hours), or urokinase (4,400 U/kg/hr infusion over 12 hours).

- Unfractionated heparin is given at the same time with PTT goal 1.5 to 2.0 times control.

Surgical: Immediate surgical consultation is warranted especially in the setting of acute heart failure

CCU Tip: Any patient with prosthetic cardiac valve who is admitted to the intensive care unit with heart failure, stroke, fever, or other thromboembolic events should have an extensive evaluation of heart valves, including a TTE and in most cases a TEE.

thrombosis is 2% to 4% per year and occurs with equal frequency in both bioprosthetic valves and mechanical valves despite adequate anticoagulation (Fig. 13.3). Increased risk occurs with mitral prostheses, atrial fibrillation, and subtherapeutic anticoagulation. Pannus formation, caused

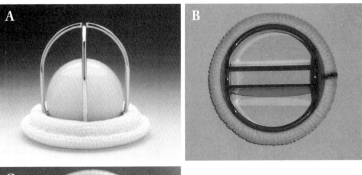

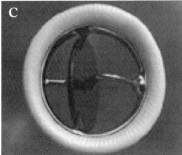

FIGURE 13.1. Mechanical valves include (A) caged-ball valves (Starr-Edwards), (B) bileaflet-tilting-disk valves (St. Jude Medical, Carbomedics), and (C) single-tilting-disk valves (Bjork-Shiley, Medtronic-Hall).

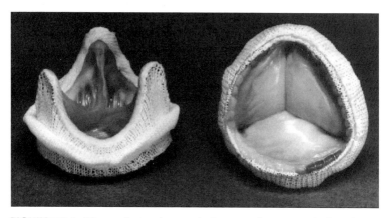

FIGURE 13.2. Bioprosthetic valves can be heterografts composed of porcine or bovine tissue typically mounted on a stent to which the leaflets and sewing ring are attached (i.e., Carpentier-Edwards).

by fibrous tissue ingrowth, is a less common cause of prosthetic valve dysfunction (Fig. 13.4). Additionally, pannus formation can occur in combination with thrombus.

Presentation

The clinical presentation is typically acute including heart failure, dyspnea, signs of poor perfusion, or systemic embolization. Other patients, however, can have a more subacute course spanning days to weeks.

Diagnostic Tests

All patients with suspected prosthetic valve obstruction should undergo transthoracic echocardiography (TTE) or transesophageal echocardiography (TEE) if adequate visualization is not obtained. Decreased movement of the disk, increased transvalvular gradient, thrombus itself, and regurgitation can be seen. Distinguishing thrombus from pannus is difficult but in general, thrombus tends to be more mobile and less echo dense, and is associated with spontaneous echo contrast. Pannus is highly echogenic and is firmly fixed to the valvular apparatus. Cinefluoroscopy is a simple adjunctive tool to assess disk motion for mechanical valves and valve ring stability.

Treatment

If valve obstruction is due to pannus formation, treatment is surgical replacement as fibrinolysis is ineffective. However, valve thrombosis is

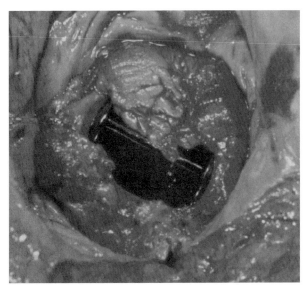

FIGURE 13.3. Valve thrombosis.

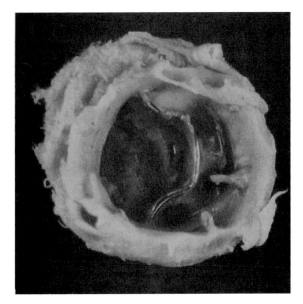

FIGURE 13.4. Tissue overgrowth on a prosthetic valve.

treated with anticoagulation with intravenous heparin. If the thrombus is nonobstructive and less than 5 mm, it is often appropriate to treat with anticoagulation alone. Patients should be monitored by TEE for close surveillance of thrombus size and for development of obstruction. For obstructive thrombosis, treatment strategies are valve replacement, thrombectomy, or fibrinolysis. However, replacement is favored over thrombectomy due to a lower rate of recurrent thrombosis. In the case of left-sided thrombosis, surgery is the preferred mode because of risk of systemic embolization with fibrinolysis. Emergent surgery is indicated for those with large clot burden or those with NYHA functional class III–IV heart failure. Mortality with surgery is approximately 15% and may reach 69% depending on severity of New York Heart Association (NYHA) functional class and need for emergency surgery.

Fibrinolysis is considered the treatment of choice for patients with right-sided valve thrombosis and is reserved for patients who are hemodynamically unstable, have a high operative risk, or have other contraindications for surgery. Successful fibrinolysis is achieved in approximately 70% of patients.

Fibrinolysis should be avoided in the following settings: (Adopted from ACC/AHA 2006 Valve guidelines)

- Active internal bleeding
- History of hemorrhagic stroke
- Recent trauma or neoplasm
- Diabetic hemorrhagic retinopathy
- Large thrombi
- Mobile thrombi
- Severe hypertension (>200/120 mmHg)
- Hypotension or shock
- NYHA class III–IV

Approved fibrinolytic regimens include alteplase (10 mg bolus, then 90 mg over 90 minutes), streptokinase (500,000 IU over 20 minutes, and then 1.5 MIU over 10 hours), or urokinase (4,400 U/kg/hr infusion over 12 hours). Unfractionated heparin is given at the same time (PTT goal 1.5 to 2.0 times control) when using alteplase. Duration of fibrinolytic therapy depends on resolution of gradients and improvement of valve area by Doppler echocardiography and should be stopped if there is no hemodynamic improvement in 24 hours or incomplete hemodynamic improvement after 72 hours. If fibrinolysis is successful, IV heparin should be continued until INR reaches 3 to 4 for aortic prostheses and 3.5 to 4.5 for valves in the mitral position.

Low dose aspirin should be added if not being taken already. If partially successful, subcutaneous heparin twice daily can be used to achieve PTT 55 to 80 seconds with INR goal 2.5 to 3.5 for 3 months.

EMBOLIZATION

Background
Systemic embolization in patients with prosthetic valves results from valve thrombosis, vegetations, left atrial thrombus, or rarely from embolization of portion of the prosthesis itself. The annual risk ranges from 1% to 2% despite therapeutic anticoagulation and is similar in patients with bioprosthetic valves and those with mechanical valves who are receiving adequate anticoagulation. The risk is greater for valves in the mitral position, caged-ball valves, and multiple prosthetic valves. It is also greater during the first few weeks to months after implantation before the valve is fully endothelialized. Other risk factors for embolic events include age >70, atrial fibrillation, left-ventricular (LV) dysfunction, hypercoagulable state, and prior thromboembolic events.

Presentation
Most cases of left-sided prosthetic valve embolic events present as cerebrovascular insults. The patient may present with stigmata of embolization to other organs including extremities, bowel, and kidney. In the case of right-sided prosthetic valves, the patient may present with signs and symptoms consistent with pulmonary embolus.

Diagnostic Tests
Evaluation includes TEE to evaluate for potential valve thrombosis and clinically excluding infective endocarditis.

Treatment
Anticoagulation therapy should be stopped and evaluation for intracerebral hemorrhage be undertaken following a cerebral embolic event. Anticoagulation can be considered in 72 hours with intravenous heparin at a lower PTT goal (40–50 seconds) depending on size of infarct and systemic arterial pressure. If embolization occurred to other solid organs, anticoagulation should be continued. If an embolic event occurred while on adequate therapy, the INR goal is increased by 0.5 (e.g., previous goal INR 2 to 3 is now 2.5 to 3.5) and ASA 80 to 100 mg/day is added if not previously on ASA. If previously on ASA alone, the dose should be increased to 325 mg/day and the addition of warfarin with a goal INR 2 to 3 can be considered.

ACUTE MANAGEMENT

Diagnostic Tests:

- **CXR:** Not very helpful
- **TTE:** Should evaluate
  - disk movement
  - transvalvular gradient
  - presence of thrombus
- **TEE:** Is frequently necessary for suspected prosthetic valve embolization:
  - in addition to above TTE features
  - differentiate thrombus from endocarditis or pannus

Cinefluoroscopy:

- To assess disk motion and opening and closing angles

Management:

- **Tools:** May need pulmonary artery catheter for hemodynamic assessment
- Arterial line, IV access
- **STAT labs:** CBC, CMP, PT, INR, PTT, type and screen, blood cultures

Medications:

- IV heparin for 72 hours with intravenous heparin at a lower PTT goal (40–50 seconds).
- If an embolic event occurred while on adequate therapy, the INR goal is increased by 0.5
- Aspirin 80 to 100 mg/day is added if not previously on ASA.
- If previously on ASA alone, the dose should be increased to 325 mg/day
- Consider adding warfarin with a goal INR of 2 to 3

Surgical: Within immediate surgical consultation is warranted especially if large thrombus is present.

CCU Tip: Obtain immediate TTE and TEE for any patient with a prosthetic valve who presents with an embolic event.

STRUCTURAL FAILURE

Background

Structural failure of mechanical valves is exceedingly rare with the exception of the Bjork-Shiley convexoconcave single-tilting-disk, which was withdrawn after reports of strut fracture and disk migration. In contrast, bioprosthetic valves are less durable and will eventually fail. Potential

---

ACUTE MANAGEMENT

Diagnostic Tests:

- **CXR:** Not very helpful
- **TTE:** Should evaluate
  - disk movement
  - transvalvular gradient
  - presence of thrombus
  - valve dehiscence
- **TEE:** Is frequently necessary for suspected prosthetic valve dysfunction:
  - in addition to above TTE features
  - assess physiologic function

Cinefluoroscopy:

- To assess disk motion and opening and closing angles
- To assess outlet-strut separation without complete strut fracture
- To determine the portion of valve that has embolized

Management:

- **Tools:** May need pulmonary artery catheter for hemodynamic assessment
- Arterial line, IV access
- **STAT labs:** CBC, CMP, PT, INR, PTT, type, and screen

Medications:

- Hemodynamic management for congestive heart failure

Surgical: Immediate surgical consultation is warranted.

causes of bioprosthetic valve failure include valve tear or rupture of valve cusp from calcification, valvular stenosis, immunological rejection, mechanical stress, and endocarditis. It is more common in younger patients, especially those less than 40 years of age and those with mitral prostheses.

Presentation

The clinical presentation of strut fracture of mechanical valves is usually catastrophic with loss of consciousness and hemodynamic collapse. In the aortic position, patients with strut fracture die within minutes but those with mitral-valve prostheses may survive long enough to undergo surgery. Structural failure in bioprosthetic valves is associated with progressive symptoms of heart failure due to valvular regurgitation or stenosis.

Diagnostic Tests

Valvular regurgitation or stenosis is assessed by TTE and/or TEE. Cinefluoroscopy can be used to diagnose patients with mechanical valves that have outlet-strut separation without complete strut fracture.

Treatment

Treatment of prosthetic valvular structural failure is surgical replacement.

ENDOCARDITIS

Background

The cumulative risk of prosthetic valve endocarditis is 3% to 6% with the greatest risk in the first 3 months postoperatively. Early infection (within the first 2 months after valve replacement) results from perioperative bacteremia either from direct intraoperative contamination or hematogenous spread in the early weeks post surgery. The pathogens are usually coagulase-negative staphylococci, followed by S. aureus, gram-negative bacilli, enterococci, and fungi. After 2 months, the pathogens are similar to those found in native valve endocarditis, most often streptococci. Mortality for early prosthetic valve endocarditis is 30% to 80% whereas late infection (after 2 months) has a mortality rate of 20% to 40%.

Presentation

Common presentations of patients with prosthetic valve endocarditis include fever, anorexia, decompensated heart failure, heart block, and systemic embolization. On exam, there may be a new or different murmur. Patients with early endocarditis rarely present with peripheral stigmata including Roth spots, Osler's nodes, or Janeway lesions. They can, however, present with a fulminant course characterized by hypoperfusion and shock. Myocardial infarction or sudden death are less common presentations.

Diagnostic Tests

Blood cultures should be obtained immediately, preferably before antibiotic therapy is started. All patients with suspected infective endocarditis should undergo echocardiography, with both TTE and TEE. Although TEE is more sensitive in detecting small vegetations, paravalvular abscesses, paravalvular leak, and fistulae, it may not be able to completely visualize the aortic valve. Negative echocardiography, however, does not exclude prosthetic valve endocarditis especially if clinical suspicion is high. A repeat study should be considered after an interval.

Treatment

Broad-spectrum antibiotics should be instituted in patients with suspected prosthetic valve endocarditis and tailored once speciation and sensitivities are known. Approximately half of patients with streptococcal endocarditis will be cured with IV antibiotics alone. Patients must be monitored for signs of progressive CHF, conduction abnormalities, and development of annular abscess, fistulae, or paravalvular leak. Treatment of prosthetic valve endocarditis with medical therapy alone is frequently ineffective. In general, infection with organisms other than streptococcus usually requires valve replacement. **Indications for surgical therapy of prosthetic valve endocarditis include**

- Early prosthetic valve endocarditis
- Heart failure with prosthetic valve dysfunction
- Fungal endocarditis
- Staphylococcal endocarditis not responding to antibiotic therapy
- Evidence of paravalvular leak, annular or aortic abscess, sinus or aortic true-or-false aneurysm, fistula, new-onset conduction disturbance
- Infection with gram-negative organisms or organisms with poor response to antibiotic therapy
- Recurrent peripheral emboli despite therapy
- Patients who have been on warfarin should have the warfarin discontinued and started on heparin in preparation for possible surgery. Again, if a cerebrovascular embolic event has occurred, heparin should be discontinued until intracranial hemorrhage has been excluded by CT or MRI. Last, aspirin should be stopped if it is part of an antithrombotic regimen in anticipation of surgery.

PARAVALVULAR LEAK AND HEMOLYSIS

Background

Paravalvular leak is an uncommon complication that is most often associated with infective endocarditis and infrequently with improper insertion of the prosthesis. It may be associated with hemolysis and anemia from high shear stress and turbulence.

Presentation

With mild paravalvular leak, patients may be asymptomatic. With moderate to severe leak, patients can present with symptoms of heart failure and anemia.

Diagnosis

Echocardiography can identify regurgitant jets of high shear stress or abnormal "rocking" of the prosthesis. Cinefluoroscopy may also identify valve ring instability. Blood cultures should be obtained to rule out infective endocarditis. Lactate dehydrogenase, haptoglobin, reticulocyte count, total and direct bilirubin, and a peripheral blood smear should be obtained to evaluate hemolysis.

Treatment

Mild paravalvular leak in and of itself is not an indication for surgery. These patients can be observed with serial echocardiograms. Mild hemolysis can be treated with folate and iron supplementation and tight blood pressure control to decrease shear stress. Patients with more severe leaks, CHF, or anemia requiring repeated transfusions require valvular repair or replacement. If the paravalvular leak is a result of endocarditis, then treatment should be as previously outlined with intravenous antibiotics and valve replacement.

CLINICAL TIPS

- Cinefluoroscopy is a simple, but often overlooked, imaging modality that can give useful information especially in mechanical valves.
- Unexplained fever in a patient with a prosthetic valve is endocarditis until proven otherwise.
- Culture-negative endocarditis most often results from recent antibiotic treatment, fungal endocarditis, or endocarditis due to fastidious organisms such as the HACEK group (Haemophilus, Actinobacillus, Cardiobacterium, Eikenella, Kingella). Blood cultures should be held for extended incubation for fastidious organisms or appropriate PCR assay.

ACUTE MANAGEMENT

Diagnostic Tests:

- **CXR:** Not very helpful
- **ECG:** Assess for conduction abnormalities
- **TTE:** Should evaluate
  - disk movement
  - regurgitant jet
  - paravalvular leak
  - transvalvular gradient
- **TEE:** Is frequently necessary for suspected prosthetic paravalvular leak and hemolysis
  - in addition to above TTE features
  - assess regurgitant jets of high shear stress or abnormal "rocking" of the prosthesis
  - rule out perivalvular abscess formation

Cinefluoroscopy:

- To assess valve ring instability

Management:

- **Tools:** May need pulmonary artery catheter for hemodynamic assessment
- Arterial line, IV access
- **STAT labs:** CBC, CMP, PT, INR, PTT, lactate dehydrogenase, haptoglobin, reticulocyte count, total and direct bilirubin, peripheral blood smear, type and screen, blood cultures

Medications:

- Mild hemolysis can be treated with folate and iron supplementation and tight blood pressure control to decrease shear stress
- Severe leaks with congestive heart failure or anemia requiring repeated transfusions will need valvular repair or replacement.
- In general, patients should be treated with PRBC, folate, and iron supplementation
- Afterload reduction with nitroprusside may be necessary
- Consider dopamine in rare cases where paravalvular leakage is very severe and patients present with hypotension

Surgical: Immediate surgical consultation is warranted.

DISCHARGE

Almost all patients presenting with prosthetic valve complications require ICU observation until a definitive therapeutic plan is established. Once clinically stable and after the underlying pathology has been corrected, transfer to telemetry floor under close monitoring can be considered.

RECOMMENDED READING

1. Bonow RO, et al. ACC/AHA guidelines for the management of patients with valvular heart disease. *Circulation.* August 1, 2006; 114(5):e84–231.
2. Vongpatanasin W, Hillis LD, Lange RA. Prosthetic heart valves. *N Engl J Med.* 1996; 335:407–416.
3. Lengyel M, Fuster V, Keltai M, et al. Guidelines for management of left-sided prosthetic valve thrombosis: a role for thrombolytic therapy: Consensus Conference on Prosthetic Valve Thrombosis. *J Am Coll Cardiol.* 1997; 30:1521–1526.
4. Karchmer, AW. *In Principles and Practice of Infectious Diseases.* Philadelphia, PA: Mandell; 2000:903.

Arrhythmias

CHAPTER 14

Narrow Complex Tachycardia

ROSS A. DOWNEY

Narrow complex tachycardia (NCT) is a common clinical problem that is defined as an arrhythmia with a rate faster than 100 bpm and a QRS duration of ≤120 msec. Nearly all NCTs are supraventricular in origin and require atrial and/or atrioventricular junctional tissue for their maintenance. The most common mechanistic cause of NCTs is reentry. Increased automaticity and triggered activity account for the remainder.

PRESENTATION

NCTs are common, frequently repetitive, occasionally sustained, but rarely life threatening in patients with structurally normal hearts. Patients are often asymptomatic but can present with palpitations, fatigue, lightheadedness, chest discomfort, dyspnea, presyncope or frank syncope. However, cardiac intensive care unit (CICU) patients frequently have underlying heart disease and any NCT may have significant hemodynamic consequences requiring a prompt intervention. The patient's clinical history of arrhythmia-related symptoms regarding the number of episodes, duration, frequency, mode of onset, and possible triggers often yield important clues as to the type of NCT present.

PHYSICAL EXAMINATION

The physical examination should be directed at assessing clinical stability and identifying associated cardiac disease and exacerbating factors as it rarely leads to a definitive diagnosis.

ACUTE MANAGEMENT

Diagnostic Tests:

- **ECG:** A 12-lead ECG is the critical first step.
- **Vagal Maneuvers:** May be useful in the setting of regular supraventricular tachycardias. Press gently on the carotid artery near the bifurcation of the internal and external carotids; typically located at the level of the jaw.
- **Adenosine:** 6 mg IV push, followed by 12 mg IV push. Always use an IV as proximal to the heart as possible.

Management:

- **Tools:** Two large-bore IV lines, defibrillator
- **STAT labs:** Basic metabolic profile, magnesium

Medications:

- Adenosine 6 mg IV push, followed by 12 mg IV push
- Amiodarone 150 mg IV bolus followed by 1 mg/min for 6 hours and 0.5 mg/min for 18 hours
- Metoprolol 5 mg IV every 5 min, followed by mouth dosing
- Verapamil 5–10 mg IV over 2 minutes
- Diltiazem 20 mg IV over 2 minutes, followed by a drip

CCU Tip:

The most important clinical decision acutely is assessing the patient's stability. If the patient is deemed unstable as a consequence of the narrow complex tachycardia, immediate synchronized DC cardioversion (DCC) with appropriate sedation is indicated. Signs of instability include hypotension, heart failure or pulmonary congestion, shortness of breath, shock, decreased level of consciousness, angina, or acute myocardial infarction, or other end-organ damage.

DIFFERENTIAL DIAGNOSIS

- Sinus tachycardia (ST)
- Inappropriate sinus tachycardia (IST)
- Sinus node reentrant tachycardia (SNRT)
- Atrial tachycardia (AT)

- Multifocal atrial tachycardia (MAT)
- Atrial fibrillation (Afib)
- Atrial flutter (Aflutter)
- Atrioventricular nodal reentrant tachycardia (AVNRT)
- Atrioventricular reentrant tachycardia (orthodromic AVRT)
- Focal junctional tachycardia (FJT)
- Nonparoxysmal junctional tachycardia (NPJT)

RISK FACTORS

- Age/Hypertension
- Primary electrical disorders/Electrolyte imbalance
- CAD/history of myocardial infarction (MI) or myocardial scarring/ Cardiac ischemia
- Congestive heart failure (CHF)/Cardiomyopathy
- Chronic pulmonary disease/ pulmonary embolism (PE)/Hypoxia
- Hyperthyroidism/Pheochromocytoma
- Congenital heart disease/Valvular disease
- Sepsis/Shock/Hyperthermia
- Illicit drugs/Toxins/Caffeine/Alcohol

DIAGNOSTIC TESTS

General Approach
The 12-lead ECG is the primary diagnostic test. The resting 12-lead ECG should be assessed for the following: rhythm, pre-excitation (delta wave), prolonged QT interval, segment abnormalities, or evidence of underlying heart disease.

A 12-lead ECG taken during the NCT should be assessed using the following criteria:

Regularity of Rhythm
Regular
– ST/IST/SNRT/AT/Aflutter/AVNRT/AVRT/FJT/NPJT
Regularly Irregular
– *AT, *Aflutter (*with variable block)
Irregularly Irregular
Afib, MAT, occasionally FJT

*A running 12-lead ECG at the time adenosine administration is very helpful to diagnose and document the particular arrhythmia

Atrial Activity (Regular NCT)
Atrial rate > ventricular rate
– Aflutter, AT
Short RP interval (RP shorter than PR)
– AVNRT, AVRT, AT (with AV delay)
Long RP interval
– AT, PJRT, AVNRT (atypical)
Normal P-wave morphology
– ST, SNRT, IST
Abnormal P-wave morphology
– Retrograde: ANVRT, AVRT, PJRT, AT (low atrial origin)
Atypical: AT, Aflutter ("saw-tooth" pattern)

Response to Adenosine or Vagal Maneuvers (Regular NCT)
No response
– Inadequate delivery/dose and VT (fascicular or high septal origin)
Gradual slowing and reacceleration of rate
– ST, AT, & FJT
Sudden termination
– AVNRT, AVRT, SNRT, and AT
Persisting atrial tachycardia with transient AV block
– Aflutter and AT

Determining the likely mechanism responsible for the supraventricular tachycardia is often useful in helping to narrow the differential diagnosis. Each of the following three mechanisms display characteristic properties.

Reentry is the most common mechanism and is characterized by a paroxysmal nature with abrupt onset and termination often in association with a premature beat. Reentry is very susceptible to adenosine, vagal maneuvers, and direct current cardioversion (DCC) and able to be reproducibly induced and terminated with programmed stimulation.

Automaticity typically has a "warm-up" and "warm-down" period when the arrhythmia begins and ends, manifested as acceleration and slowing of the tachycardia. It is often seen in acutely ill patients under metabolic stressful conditions. They do not respond to adenosine or vagal maneuvers outside of temporary slowing of AV conduction. DCC is generally not effective as the arrhythmias tend to recur promptly and the arrhythmias are less likely to be induced or terminated by programmed pacing techniques.

Triggered activity has some features of both reentry and increased automaticity. Like automaticity, triggered activity involves positive ions leaking into the cardiac cells, which create afterdepolarizations. If enough afterpolarizations occur, a new action potential is generated. It also often displays a warm-up and warm-down period. Unlike automaticity but similar to reentry, triggered activity is not always spontaneous and can be induced by premature beats/programmed pacing techniques. This arrhythmia mechanism is usually seen in the setting of drug toxicity or metabolic abnormalities.

Specific Diagnosis

Sinus Tachycardia (ST)
Considered a normal response to a myriad of physiologically stressful conditions. ST normally increases and decreases in rate gradually (warm-up and cool-down pattern) rather than in an abrupt paroxysmal fashion. ST, inappropriate sinus tachycardia (IST), and sinus node reentrant tachycardia (SNRT) all have normal P-wave axis and morphology given their mutually shared origination from the SA node and/or perinodal tissue. (Automaticity)

Inappropriate Sinus Tachycardia (IST)
A condition in which patients' resting heart rate is abnormally high (greater than 100 bpm), increases rapidly with minimal exertion, and is accompanied by symptoms of palpitations, fatigue, and exercise intolerance. The mechanism and primary etiology of IST are unclear. No formal diagnostic criteria exist and therefore, the diagnosis is one primarily of exclusion after the other causes of ST are excluded. (Intrinsic SN dysfunction vs. dysautonomia)

Sinus Node Reentrant Tachycardia (SNRT)
Abrupt onset and termination (paroxysmal nature) along with its ability to be induced and terminated by pacing distinguish it from ST and IST. (Reentry)

Atrial Tachycardia (AT)
Characterized by regular atrial activation from a single focus at rates between 100 to 250 bpm. All three mechanisms likely can cause AT resulting in a varied manner of presentations. AT usually, but not always, is a long RP arrhythmia with an isoelectric baseline between P waves (unlike Aflutter) that are of different morphology from those arising

from the SN (unlike SN originating arrhythmias). (Reentry/Automaticity/ Triggered)

Multifocal atrial tachycardia (MAT)
An irregularly irregular rhythm characterized by at least three different P-wave morphologies, with the P waves separated by isoelectric intervals and associated with varying P-P, R-R, and PR intervals. (Automaticity)

Atrial Fibrillation (Afib)
By far the most common NCT encountered in CICU patients. Afib is an irregularly irregular rhythm characterized by continuous and chaotic atrial fibrillatory activity at a rate of 350 to 600 impulses/minute without the presence of distinct P waves. (Reentry)

Atrial Flutter (Aflutter)
Usually a regular SVT but occasionally can be regularly irregular secondary to variable AV block. Common/typical Aflutter is a macroreentrant arrhythmia that travels in a circular counterclockwise direction in the right atrium at approximately 300 impulses/minute that characteristically produces flutter waves (saw tooth) most evident in the inferior leads. The use of adenosine can often unmask the underlying characteristic atrial activity. (Reentry)

Atrioventricular Nodal Reentrant Tachycardia (AVNRT)
The most common regular paroxysmal NCT. It involves reciprocation between two functionally and anatomically distinct pathways in the AV node and/or perinodal atrial tissue that have different conduction and refractory properties. In typical AVNRT (90%–95%), the slow pathway serves as the anterograde limb and the fast pathway serves as the retrograde limb. This usually results in a short RP interval (≤70 ms) and often with a pseudo-r' in lead V1. (Reentry)

Atrioventricular Reentrant Tachycardia (AVRT)
The second most common regular paroxysmal NCT. It involves reciprocation between the AV node and an **extra** nodal accessory pathway(s) that connect the atrium and the ventricle. Accessory pathways are classified according to their location, type of conduction (decremental or no), and direction of conduction (anterograde, retrograde, or both). Pathways that are capable of anterograde conduction (manifest) can demonstrate pre-excitation on an ECG (delta wave). AVRT is also subclassified according to the direction of the macroreentry circuit: (a) orthodromic (down the AV node and up the accessory pathway), (b) and antidromic

(down the accessory pathway and up the AV node, which results is a wide complex SVT). AVRT is usually orthodromic (90%–95%) and characterized by a short RP interval except the permanent junctional reciprocating tachycardia (PJRT) variety. There is variable evidence of pre-excitation at baseline depending on whether the accessory pathway can conduct in an anterograde direction. Wolff-Parkinson-White (WPW) syndrome requires the presence of **both** pre-excitation on ECG and tachyarrhythmias. (Reentry)

Focal Junctional Tachycardia (FJT)

A very uncommon arrhythmia that comprises several distinct clinical syndromes with a unifying feature of their origin from the AV node or His bundle. It is most common in children and younger adults, is usually exercise or stress related, has heart-rate ranges between 110 to 250 bpm, and AV dissociation is often present. (Automaticity/Triggered)

Nonparoxysmal Junctional Tachycardia (NPJT)

A benign arrhythmia in itself, but may be a marker for a serious underlying condition. It typically displays a warm-up and cool-down pattern and commonly is in one-to-one AV association at rates 70 to 120 bpm. Often, the clinical setting and ECG findings together can help establish the diagnosis. (Automaticity/Triggered)

MEDICAL MANAGEMENT

General Measures

Acute therapy includes immediate cardioversion in hemodynamically unstable patients and vagal maneuvers and specific pharmacologic therapy for NCT based on the ECG/mechanistic diagnosis. **Reentry** arrhythmias involving the AV node are particularly susceptible to adenosine and vagal maneuvers. **Automaticity** arrhythmias are best managed by treating the underlying conditions/disease process. DCC is generally not recommended because of the likelihood of prompt recurrence. **Triggered** arrhythmias should be screened for whether digitalis toxicity is the inciting cause.

Specific Measures

Sinus Tachycardia (ST)

Assess and treat other precipitating factors (temperature, infection, hypovolemia, pain, anxiety, anemia, etc).

Inappropriate Sinus Tachycardia (IST)

Beta blockers, calcium channel blockers, and type 1c antiarrhythmic agents constitute the mainstay of treatment for IST. Given the heterogeneous symptoms and response to treatment, other treatment modalities are often employed.

Sinus Node Reentrant Tachycardia (SNRT)

Most episodes require no specific therapy since the usual rates (100–150 bpm) rarely produce hemodynamic compromise. Vagal maneuvers are particularly effective given the extensive autonomic innervation of the SA node. Adenosine can acutely terminate SNRT and beta blockers, verapamil, amiodarone, and digoxin can also be used to terminate and/or slow the rate.

Atrial Tachycardia (AT)

No large trials have been conducted, but the mainstay of acute treatment usually is IV beta blockers or calcium channel blockers to (a) convert the patient (rare) and (b) more likely achieve rate control through slowing conducting in the AV node. Direct suppression of the AT focus may be attempted with class 1A, 1C, or III medications. Given the variety of causal mechanisms, treatments should be tailored to the most likely underlying mechanism when possible.

Multifocal Atrial Tachycardia (MAT)

The most effective therapy in MAT is aimed at the inciting underlying disease. This includes treating pulmonary and cardiac disease, hypokalemia, and hypomagnesemia. Beta blockers and verapamil have been shown to be beneficial but antiarrhythmics and DCC are not effective in treating MAT.

Atrial Fibrillation (Afib)

There are three main treatment issues: (1) rhythm control, (2) ventricular rate control, and (3) thromboembolic prevention. Rhythm control concerns whether to restore sinus rhythm or leave the patient in Afib. Patients rendered unstable by Afib are candidates for immediate DCC. Stable patients in Afib <48 hours can be either chemically/electrically cardioverted or simply rate controlled while in Afib. The decision to cardiovert and what is considered optimal rate control depends on the patient's situation. IV/by mouth beta blockers, calcium channel blockers, and digoxin are the agents most commonly used to obtain adequate rate control. Amiodarone is also used as it provides some rate control (especially IV) and is effective in keeping people in sinus rhythm. Only higher dose (>1,500 mg/day IV) amiodarone is superior to placebo in converting recent-onset Afib to sinus rhythm. Stable patients in Afib >48 hours, for whom restoration of sinus rhythm is desired, should either have a TEE to rule out intracardiac thrombus or 3 weeks of therapeutic anticoagulation prior to cardioversion to minimize their risk of thromboembolism. Almost all CICU patients who are in Afib >48 hours or of unclear duration should be anticoagulated unless contraindicated. Alternatively, patients with "lone" Afib and low-risk patients may be treated with 325 mg of aspirin daily. A clinical prediction rule (CHADS) was developed for estimating risk for stroke in patients with atrial fibrillation based on five risk factors: **C**ongestive heart failure (active within the past 100 days or documented by echocardiography), **H**ypertension (systolic or diastolic), **A**ge ≥75, **D**iabetes mellitus, and history of **S**troke or transient ischemic attack (TIA). Each risk factor is assigned one point except for history of stroke or TIA, which is assigned two points for a total of six points. A score of 0 to 1 was designated low risk, 2 to 3 moderate risk, and 4 to 6 high risk.

Atrial Flutter (Aflutter)

Aflutter is a reentry arrhythmia that is independent of the SA and AV node for its activity and as such, usually is not terminated by adenosine and/or vagal maneuvers. Patients with Aflutter commonly have episodes of Afib; therefore, both arrhythmias share the same general issues and are treated in a similar manner. Rate control is generally more difficult to achieve with Aflutter than with Afib.

Atrioventricular Nodal Reentrant Tachycardia (AVRNT)

Given AVNRT's dependence on the AV node, treatments that block or slow conduction in the AV node are helpful. Vagal maneuvers and adenosine are particularly effective in terminating AVNRT. Intravenous calcium channel blockers and beta blockers are also effective.

Atrioventricular Reentrant Tachycardia (AVRT)

Orthodromic AVRT normally presents as a narrow complex artachycardia (NCT) and antidromic AVRT always as a wide complex tachycardia (WCT). Both types of AVRT are AV node-dependent and thus respond to AV nodal-blocking therapies. While it is reasonable to use AV nodal blocking medications acutely in patients presenting with narrow complex AVRT (immediate synchronized DCC should be available should the rhythm degenerate), it is not safe in patients when they present with WCT. Patients with accessory pathways can present with WCTs resulting from (1) orthodromic AVRT with aberrant conduction, (2) antidromic AVRT or, most importantly, (3) atrial arrhythmias (AT/Aflutter/Afib) with anterograde conduction down an accessory pathway. Since it is often initially impossible to tell the mechanism of WCTs in patients with an accessory pathway, they should be treated with agents that slow conduction in the accessory pathways (procainamide, flecainide, sotalol, or amiodarone). Since atrial arrhythmias with anterograde accessory pathway conduction are **not** AV node dependent, AV nodal blocking therapies are ineffective and potentially very dangerous. Beta blockers, calcium channel blockers, digoxin, and adenosine should be avoided in patients presenting with WCTs as they may encourage preferential conduction down accessory pathways and accelerate ventricular rates, precipitating ventricular fibrillation (VF). Adenosine, although effective in treating orthodromic and antidromic AVRT, may induce Afib in up to 15% of cases and should therefore be used with caution. In patients with WPW syndrome, Afib is a potentially life-threatening arrhythmia, especially when the accessory pathway

CLINICAL PRESENTATION TIPS

- Assess the patients' stability in context of their tachycardia.
- Compare present ECG with old ECGs when possible.
- History can often be revealing.
- Atrial tachycardia with atrioventricular block, think digitalis toxicity.
- Regular narrow complex tachycardia without discernable P waves, think atrioventricular nodal reentrant tachycardia.
- Tachycardia termination with a P wave after the last QRS complex favors atrioventricular reentry tachycardia or atrioventricular nodal reentrant tachycardia.

has a short anterograde refractory period capable of rapid ventricular conduction. Again, immediate synchronize DCC is appropriate for unstable patients.

Focal Junctional Tachycardia (FJT)

Little is known regarding the pharmacological therapy of FJT. Drug therapy is variably successful with beta blockers and IV flecainide having been used to slow or terminate FJT in some patients. Catheter ablation can be curative but carries a 5% to 10% risk of AV block.

Nonparoxysmal Junctional Tachycardia (NPJT)

The mainstay of treatment of NPJT is correction of the underlying abnormality. Associated conditions include digitalis toxicity, postcardiac surgery, hypokalemia, myocardial ischemia or inflammation, and chronic obstructive pulmonary disease (COPD) with hypoxia. Withholding digitalis is usually sufficient when NPJT is the only sign of toxicity. Digitalis-binding agents may be indicated if ventricular arrhythmias or high-grade heart block is noted. Beta blockers and calcium channel blockers can be used to suppress a persisting NPJT.

COMPLICATIONS

Hemodynamic compromise: Syncope, MI, CHF
Thromboembolic events: Especially with Afib

DISCHARGE

Patients with supraventricular tachycardias can be safely discharged from the ICU when they are hemodynamically stable. Ideally, a specific diagnosis made, precipitants identified and corrected when appropriate, and a treatment care plan formulated.

RECOMMENDED READING

1. Guidelines 2000 for cardiopulmonary resuscitation and emergency cardiovascular care. Part 6: advanced cardiovascular life support: 7D: the tachycardia algorithms. The American Heart Association in collaboration with the International Liaison Committee on Resuscitation. *Circulation.* 2000; 102:I158.
2. Blomstrom-Lundqvist, Scheinman, et al. ACC/AHA/ESC guidelines for the management of patients with supraventricular arrhythmias. 2003.
3. Fogoros RN, *Electrophysiology Testing.* 4th ed. April 2006.

CHAPTER 15

Wide-Complex Tachycardia

ADAM W. GRASSO

Wide-complex tachycardia (WCT) is defined as an arrhythmia with a rate faster than 100 beats per minute (bpm), and a QRS duration of ≥120 milliseconds (msec) on ECG or telemetry monitor. WCT may originate from a ventricular focus or may result from a supraventricular mechanism with aberrant ventricular conduction. In either of these cases, ventricular tachycardia (VT) or supraventricular tachycardia (SVT) with aberrancy, the wide QRS complex results from slower-than-normal depolarization of the ventricular myocardium. VT is commonly classified as sustained or nonsustained (<30-second duration).

PRESENTATION

Most patients with sustained WCT present with hemodynamic instability and require emergent direct current cardioversion (DCC). Symptoms can vary from mild palpitations, lightheadedness, and diaphoresis, to chest pain, syncope, shock, seizures, and cardiac arrest. WCTs can be unpredictable and frequently life threatening.

PHYSICAL EXAMINATION

- Pulselessness
- Altered mental status
- Cool clammy skin
- Hypotension
- Pulmonary edema
- Hypoxia

A C U T E MANAGEMENT

- Assess hemodynamic status!

Diagnostic Tests:

- **ECG:** To differentiate between ventricular tachycardia and supraventricular tachycardia. However, in hemodynamically unstable patients immediate DCC is essential.

Management:

- **Tools:** Two large-bore IVs for advanced cardiac life support medications, fluid resuscitation, and/or pressor agents
- **STAT labs:** CK, CKMB, Troponin, CBC, CMP, Mg, PT, INR, PTT, type and screen

Treatment:

- For witnessed collapse without telemetry monitoring, deliver precordial thump
- CPR for nonperfusing rhythms
- For VF or pulseless ventricular tachycardia, immediate unsynchronized DCC with 200 Joules (J) for a monophasic device, followed by 300J, then 360J if ventricular tachycardia persists. If a biphasic unit is being used, the sequence is 150J, 200J, 200J.
- For hemodynamically stable ventricular tachycardia, initiate advanced cardiac life support-guided drug therapy followed by synchronized DCC if pharmacologic conversion not rapidly successful
- For ischemic ventricular tachycardia, consider amiodarone (150 mg IV bolus over 10 minutes, which can be repeated, followed by 1 mg/min drip) or lidocaine (1 mg/kg bolus over 2 minutes, which can be repeated twice, followed by 2 mg/min drip).
- Correct underlying electrolyte disturbances (give magnesium sulfate 2 gm IV bolus, especially for torsades de pointes)
- Stop offending agents (i.e., drugs that increase QT interval)
- For incessant polymorphic ischemic ventricular tachycardia consider IABP, sedation, and intubation
- For clear supraventricular tachycardia with aberrancy, procainamide (15 mg/kg load at 20 mg/min, followed by 2 to 4 mg/min drip). This is the drug of choice if Wolff-Parkinson-White syndrome is present.

- In a hemodynamically stable patient, consider a beta blocker, especially in those with outflow tract ventricular tachycardia

Surgical: In rare cases, electrophysiology consultation for ablation may be indicated. In patients with ischemic ventricular tachycardia revascularization should be performed immediately.

CCU Tip: If the cause of ventricular tachycardia is bradycardia and long QT consider temporary pacemaker and/or isoproterenol (may cause ischemia and hypertension), in addition to aggressive magnesium repletion.

- Respiratory distress necessitating intubation
- Variable cannon A waves on jugular venous exam
- Variable intensity of auscultated S1
- Variable intensity of palpated pulse or arterial line pressure (>10 mmHg beat-to-beat variation)

DIFFERENTIAL DIAGNOSIS

WCTs of Ventricular Origin

Ventricular fibrillation (VF) is characterized by a chaotic, disorganized pattern of ventricular activation, which is always nonperfusing. VF is the rhythm most frequently responsible for sudden cardiac death (SCD). While it is most frequently related to coronary ischemia, VF can also result from R-on-T phenomenon, from electrical shock during the vulnerable phase of ventricular repolarization (downslope of T wave), and from degeneration of VT in the nonischemic myocardium (Fig. 15.1).

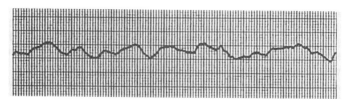

FIGURE 15.1. Representative example of ventricular fibrillation. *Source:* Waugh RA, Ramo BW, Wagner GS, et al. *Cardiac Arrhythmias: A Practical Guide for the Clinician.* 2nd ed. Philadelphia: F.A. Davis Company; 1994:204, with permission.

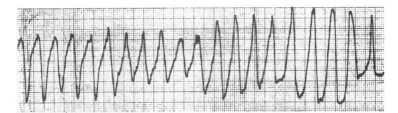

FIGURE 15.2. Torsades de pointes subtype of polymorphic ventricular tachycardia. *Source:* Waugh RA, Ramo BW, Wagner GS, et al. *Cardiac Arrhythmias: A Practical Guide for the Clinician.* 2nd ed. Philadelphia: F.A. Davis Company; 1994:278, with permission.

Polymorphic VT is also a disorganized pattern of ventricular activation, which is usually nonperfusing. The most well-known type of polymorphic VT is "torsades de pointes (TdP)," or "twisting of the points," which has a characteristic appearance (Fig. 15.2). Frequently associated with electrolyte abnormalities, namely hypokalemia and hypomagnesemia, as well as certain drugs (Table 15.1), which can prolong the QT interval, and increase the likelihood of R on T.

Monomorphic VT reflects an organized, reentrant pattern, which may or may not be associated with hemodynamic compromise (Fig. 15.3). Frequently associated with coronary ischemia or myocardial scar, it can also occur in the setting of the normal heart, as with outflow-tract VTs.

Accelerated Idioventricular Rhythm (AIVR) is a wide-complex ventricular rhythm with a rate between 60 to 100 bpm, generally associated with hemodynamic stability (Fig. 15.4). Though technically not a tachycardia, AIVR should be grouped with the WCTs, since it shares their risk factors. AIVR classically occurs during active, symptomatic coronary ischemia, as well as during the period following reperfusion therapy.

Nonsustained VT is defined as VT <30 second in duration, which may or may not be associated with hemodynamic instability (Fig. 15.5). It occurs very commonly in post-MI patients and in those with ischemic or nonischemic cardiomyopathies, as well as in normal hearts.

Ventricular tachyarrhythmias (VTA) secondary to other causes produces congenital long-QT syndrome (LQTS), which results from mutations in genes encoding myocardial ion channels and is a risk factor for polymorphic VT (TdP) in young patients with otherwise normal hearts. Brugada syndrome is another condition predisposing to VTA, which has been linked to mutations in SCN5A, the gene encoding for the

Table 15.1	Drugs linked to wide-complex tachycardia (WCT).	
Drug	Rhythm	Patient Populations at Increased Risk
Quinidine, other class Ia agents	VT, TdP	Pts on amiodarone (increased quinidine levels)
Flecainide, other class Ic agents	VT	Post-MI pts; those with hepatic or renal insufficiency, or HF.
Sotalol, Dofetilide, Ibutilide (class III)	VT, TdP	Pts on QT-prolonging drugs, with electrolyte abnormalities or renal insufficiency
Digoxin	DADs, VT (can be bidirectional)	Women, elderly, those with renal insufficiency
Phenothiazines, including anti-psychotics (chlorpromazine, thioridazine, and trifluoperazine) and anti-emetics (prochlorperazine and promethazine)	VT	Pts on other QT-prolonging drugs
Erythromycin, other macrolides	VT	Pts on other QT-prolonging drugs; with underlying HF
Cisapride (off the market in U.S.)	VT, TdP	Pts on drugs which inhibit CYP3A4
Tricyclic antidepressants (especially amitriptyline, desipramine, imipramine, nortriptyline)	VT, TdP	Pts on drugs which inhibit CYP1A2 or CYP2D6
Drugs of abuse: cocaine, amphetamines, nicotine, alcohol, inhaled glue	VT	Underlying CAD

HF, heart failure; DADs, delayed afterdepolarizations; CYP: Cytochrome P450, VT, ventricular tachycardia; TdP, torsades de pointes.

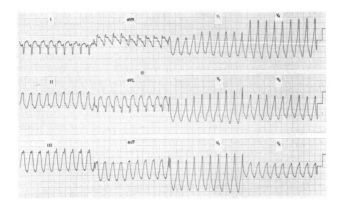

FIGURE 15.3. Monomorphic ventricular tachycardia. Note positive concordance of precordial leads. *Source:* Waugh RA, Ramo BW, Wagner GS, et al. *Cardiac Arrhythmias: A Practical Guide for the Clinician.* 2nd ed. Philadelphia: F.A. Davis Company; 1994:277, with permission.

alpha subunit of a sodium channel. This syndrome is identified by characteristic "coved" ST-segment elevations in the right precordial leads (Fig. 15.6), which are often not present at baseline, becoming unmasked by stressors such as fever or drugs. Finally, hypertrophic obstructive cardiomyopathy (HOCM), which appears to be due to mutations in

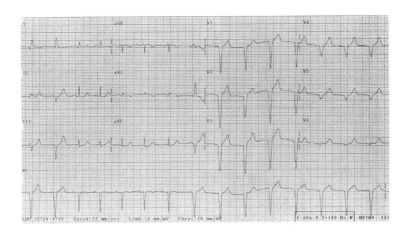

FIGURE 15.4. Accelerated idioventricular rhythm (AIVR), seen in the first two and the last eight complexes, with five intervening beats of sinus rhythm. This 12-lead ECG was performed on a 39-year-old woman with severe chest pain 2 weeks postpartum. In the cath lab she was found to have a spontaneous dissection of the LAD, requiring stenting.

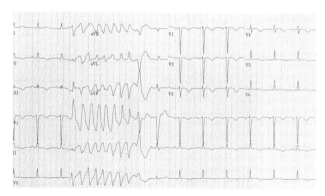

FIGURE 15.5. Nonsustained ventricular tachycardia, nine-beat run of polymorphic type, self-terminating.

myocardial structural proteins, predisposes individuals to sudden cardiac death (SCD) via VT and/or VF. Sudden collapse in young individuals, especially those with a family history of sudden death, should raise the possibility of congenital LQTS, Brugada syndrome, or HOCM.

Drugs are also a cause of VTA, most commonly through their prolongation of the QT interval. Drugs of abuse such as cocaine and amphetamines dramatically increase sympathetic outflow, and can induce VTA. Additional causes of VT include viral myocarditis (adenovirus, enterovirus, and parvovirus being most frequently implicated), inflammatory myocarditis (lymphocytic, giant cell, or granulomatous

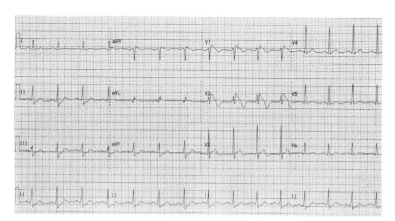

FIGURE 15.6. Brugada syndrome. Note right bundle branch block pattern and ST-segment elevation in leads V1 and V2. This ECG was performed on a 48-year-old man of Southeast Asian ancestry who had been resuscitated after sudden cardiac death.

from sarcoidosis), and arrhythmogenic right ventricular dysplasia (ARVD), a disorder of fatty infiltration of the right ventricle which predisposes to ventricular arrhythmias.

WCTs of Supraventricular Origin with Aberrant Conduction

The widened QRS in these tachyarrhythmias can be due to either aberrant conduction distal to the AV node or from ventricular pre-excitation of Wolff-Parkinson-White (WPW) syndrome.

Sinus tachycardia (ST) with a complete left or right bundle branch block (LBBB, RBBB) or a nonspecific intraventricular conduction delay (IVCD) may widen the QRS complex ≥120 msec. The conduction defect can be fixed, with a similar QRS width during normal sinus rhythm (NSR) and tachycardia, or rate-dependent, with QRS broadening as the rate increases (Fig. 15.7). Clues to the diagnosis of ST with aberrancy include conducted P waves with morphology similar to those during NSR and gradual changes in the ventricular rate.

Atrial tachycardia (AT) is similar to ST with aberrancy, except the P waves from the ectopic atrial pacemaker are generally of a different morphology from those seen during normal sinus rhythm (Fig. 15.8). Also, the onset of AT is usually of a rapid on/off nature, not gradual.

Atrial fibrillation (Afib) or atrial flutter (Aflutter)—while Afib is an irregular tachycardia, Aflutter is regular at a rate often close to 150 bpm in the case of 2 : 1 AV conduction (Figs. 15.9–15.11).

AV nodal reentrant tachycardia (AVnRT) is a very common cause of narrow-complex tachycardia. AVnRT is usually seen in patients with normal hearts, but can also occur in those with heart disease. It results from "micro-reentry," a reentrant circuit involving both fast and slow atrial pathways through the AV node. A widened QRS complex can result from the presence of an associated RBBB, LBBB, or IVCD (Fig. 15.12).

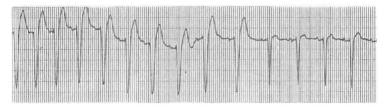

FIGURE 15.7. Sinus tachycardia with left bundle branch block. Note narrowing of QRS complex with slowing of rate. *Source:* Waugh RA, Ramo BW, Wagner GS, et al. *Cardiac Arrhythmias: A Practical Guide for the Clinician.* 2nd ed. Philadelphia: F.A. Davis Company; 1994:183, with permission.

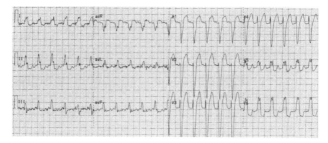

FIGURE 15.8. Atrial tachycardia with aberrant conduction (left bundle branch block morphology).

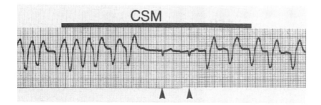

FIGURE 15.9. Atrial fibrillation with a rate-related left bundle branch block. Note resolution of bundle branch block with depressed atrioventricular conduction during carotid sinus massage (arrowheads indicate narrow QRS complexes.) *Source:* Waugh RA, Ramo BW, Wagner GS, et al. *Cardiac Arrhythmias: A Practical Guide for the Clinician.* 2nd ed. Philadelphia: F.A. Davis Company; 1994:183, with permission.

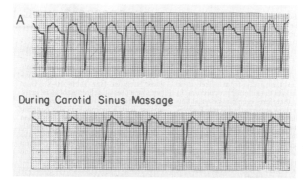

FIGURE 15.10. Atrial flutter with fixed aberrancy, ventricular rate of ~150 bpm (upper panel). Note P waves in T-wave downslopes. During carotid sinus massage (lower panel), 4:1 AV block is induced, with P waves clearly "marching" at rate of ~300 bpm. *Source:* Waugh RA, Ramo BW, Wagner GS, et al. *Cardiac Arrhythmias: A Practical Guide for the Clinician.* 2nd ed. Philadelphia: F.A. Davis Company; 1994:211, with permission.

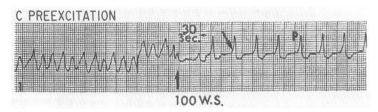

FIGURE 15.11. Atrial fibrillation with pre-excitation (Wolff-Parkinson-White syndrome), before and after 100J shock. Note delta wave (slanted arrow), P wave (P). *Source:* Waugh RA, Ramo BW, Wagner GS, et al. *Cardiac Arrhythmias: A Practical Guide for the Clinician.* 2nd ed. Philadelphia: F.A. Davis Company; 1994:167, with permission.

Antidromic AV reciprocating tachycardia (AVRT), in contrast to AVnRT, is a "macro-reentry" circuit involving an accessory pathway for AV conduction, as well as the AV node itself. In orthodromic reciprocating AVRT, a narrow complex tachycardia is seen as ventricular depolarization occurs down the AV node (and retrogradely through the accessory pathway), but a wide complex can occur secondary to aberrant ventricular conduction. In antidromic reciprocating AVRT, ventricular depolarization occurs via the accessory pathway, resulting in a wide QRS complex (Fig. 15.13). Often difficult to distinguish from VT acutely, this is a rare cause of WCT in the coronary care unit (CCU).

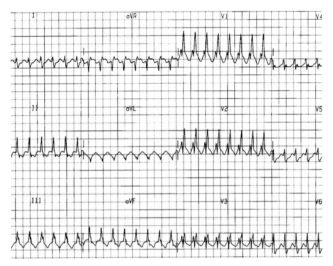

FIGURE 15.12. Atrioventricular nodal reentrant tachycardia (AVnRT) at a rate of 190 bpm, with aberrant conduction.

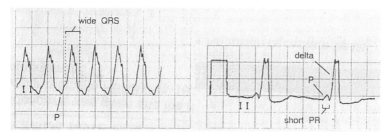

FIGURE 15.13. Antidromic atrioventricular reentry tachycardia (AVRT) at a rate of 260 bpm (left panel), and subject's ECG in sinus rhythm (right panel). Note P waves (P), short PR-interval (short PR), and delta wave (delta).

Other WCTs

Pacemaker-mediated tachycardia (PMT), although less common with today's modern pacemakers, is an endless-loop tachycardia, which can occur when VA conduction is followed by tracking of the retrograde P wave and subsequent ventricular pacing. PMT can be verified by placing a magnet over the device, which will cause VOO pacing at the backup rate and terminate the tachycardia (Fig. 15.14). PMT generally can be eliminated by lengthening the postventricular atrial refractory period (PVARP) setting of the device.

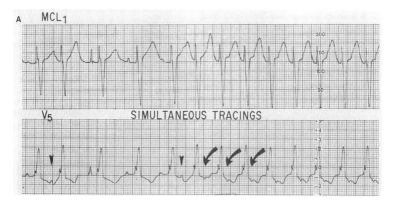

FIGURE 15.14. Pacemaker-mediated tachycardia. Fifth complex consists of a native P wave and a paced QRS (A-sense, V-pace), followed immediately by retrograde VA conduction and another P wave (arrowhead). An "endless-loop" tachycardia follows, in which ventricular pacing causes retrograde atrial activation (curved arrows), which in turn triggers pacing of the ventricle again. *Source:* Waugh RA, Ramo BW, Wagner GS, et al. *Cardiac Arrhythmias: A Practical Guide for the Clinician.* 2nd ed. Philadelphia: F.A. Davis Company; 1994:118, with permission.

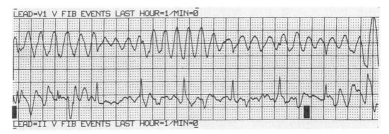

FIGURE 15.15. Atrial flutter with variable conduction (note QRS complexes on lower lead) appears to be torsades de pointes (TdP) on upper telemetry lead. Problem resolved after replacement of telemetry box and leads.

Artifactual WCT may be caused by a tremor, tooth brushing, and equipment malfunction, which can lead to the appearance of a WCT, generally seen on telemetry monitoring. Patients with artifactual WCT will usually be asymptomatic during the period of strip recording. Artifactual WCT will often not be present in all leads, with the true QRS complexes being visible marching through the period of apparent arrhythmia (Fig. 15.15). Clarification of the actual rhythm can be achieved by obtaining a 12-lead ECG, and replacing electrical equipment in the case of malfunction.

Although patients with *hypothermia* are generally not tachycardic, dramatically widened QRS complexes can be observed (Fig. 15-16).

Wide QRS complexes in *hyperkalemia* do not indicate VT, but rather a sinus rhythm with severely aberrant conduction due to the electrolyte disturbance (Fig. 15.17).

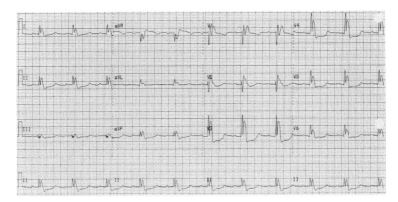

FIGURE 15-16. A patient in the emergency room with hypothermia (body temperature 31°C) had this ECG. Note the characteristic, "rabbit-eared" QRS complexes (Osborne waves), which resolved on rewarming.

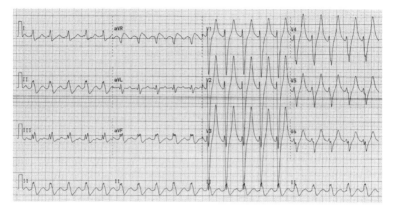

FIGURE 15.17. A 41-year-old man with end-stage renal disease on hemodialysis was admitted to the hospital with altered mental status and vague chest complaints. His initial ECG above showed a sinus tachycardia at 122 bpm, with very wide QRS complexes (180 msec) and peaked T waves. His serum potassium was found to be critically elevated at 9.2 mM.

RISK FACTORS

- Large infarct with LV dysfunction
- Ischemic and nonischemic cardiomyopathy
- Personal or family history of arrhythmias or sudden death
- Medications predisposing to VT (see Table 15.1)
- Coronary artery disease (CAD)
- Renal insufficiency, especially end-stage, on dialysis
- Cerebrovascular accident (CVA)
- Traumatic brain injury (TBI), subarachnoid hemorrhage (SAH)
- Hypothyroidism
- Anorexia nervosa
- Liquid protein or starvation diet
- Organophosphate poisoning
- Electrolyte abnormalities

DIAGNOSTIC TESTS

Laboratory findings of hypokalemia (K <3.5 mM), hypomagnesemia (Mg <1.6 mg/dL), and much less frequently, hypocalcemia (Ca <8.5 mg/dL) have been linked to the development of TdP. Hyperkalemia (K >5.0 mM, but usually higher in those with end-stage renal disease) can lead to a wide

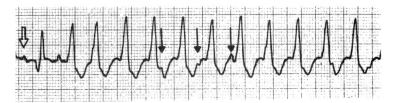

FIGURE 15.18. AV dissociation suggestive of ventricular tachycardia. Note initial P wave (open arrow), then P waves marching through, but without relationship to, the WCT (arrows). *Source:* Waugh RA, Ramo BW, Wagner GS, et al. *Cardiac Arrhythmias: A Practical Guide for the Clinician.* 2nd ed. Philadelphia: F.A. Davis Company; 1994:170, with permission.

QRS complex and a slow rate, sometimes termed a "sinoventricular" rhythm, which is really a sinus rhythm with aberrant conduction.

ECG differentiates VT from SVT (Figs. 15.18–15.20), helps locate the origin and the type of VT, which can impact treatment decision. One should also seek to obtain an old ECG, preferably showing the patient in sinus rhythm. Side-by-side comparison of old and new ECGs often can be informative regarding the origin (atrial or ventricular) of the presenting rhythm. For example, similar QRS axes would tend to suggest SVT, while markedly different axes would suggest VT. A prolonged baseline QT_C interval ($\geq$450 msec) would invoke the possibility of congenital or acquired LQTS, which would predispose the patient to ventricular arrhythmias.

Most WCTs can be classified as having either a RBBB-pattern (QRS positive in leads V1 and V2) or a LBBB-pattern (QRS negative in V1 and V2). Certain characteristics of the QRS morphology have been shown to favor VT (Fig. 15.21).

Vagal maneuvers (e.g., carotid massage) and drug administration (e.g., IV adenosine) for diagnosis, if SVT with aberrancy is suspected

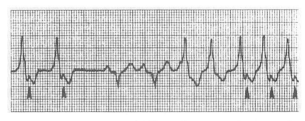

FIGURE 15.19. Ventriculoatrial (VA) conduction, with retrograde p-waves (arrowheads). *Source:* Waugh RA, Ramo BW, Wagner GS, et al. *Cardiac Arrhythmias: A Practical Guide for the Clinician.* 2nd ed. Philadelphia: F.A. Davis Company; 1994:269, with permission.

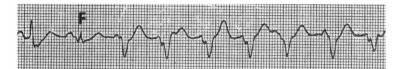

FIGURE 15.20. The first complex in this strip is sinus rhythm, while the last seven are a WCT. A fusion beat (F), resulting from collision between depolarization wavefronts originating from the sinus node and from the ventricle, strongly suggests the presence of VT. *Source:* Waugh RA, Ramo BW, Wagner GS, et al. *Cardiac Arrhythmias: A Practical Guide for the Clinician.* 2nd ed. Philadelphia: F.A. Davis Company; 1994:172, with permission.

(generally, in a young person without evidence of heart disease), are reasonable therapies in an attempt to block AV conduction and better assess atrial activity. In general, it is best to avoid calcium channel blockers or beta blockers with WCT unless the patient has a known history of SVT with aberrancy. Also, those with WPW should not be administered such agents, as they may increase the heart rate, leading to hemodynamic decompensation.

1. QRS width >0.14 s
2. Superior QRS axis
3. Morphology in precordial leads:

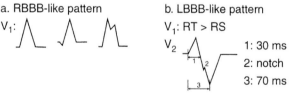

a. RBBB-like pattern

V_1:

b. LBBB-like pattern

V_1: RT > RS

V_2

1: 30 ms
2: notch
3: 70 ms

V_6: R/S ratio <1

V_6: qR

4. AV dissociation, fusion, capture present

RBBB, right bundle branch block; LBBB, left bunch branch block; AV, atrioventricular.

FIGURE 15.21. Classic morphology criteria for ventricular tachycardia. *Source:* Marso SP, Griffin BP, and Topol EJ (eds.) *Manual of Cardiovascular Medicine.* 1st ed. Philadelphia: Lippincott Williams & Wilkins; 2000:269, with permission.

Transthoracic echo (TTE) provides data on LV function and can identify areas of scarred myocardium.

MEDICAL MANAGEMENT

We cannot emphasize enough that stabilization of the unstable patient, generally achieved through DCC, should always take first priority over an in-depth diagnostic evaluation. Specific algorithms for ECG analysis have been developed to assist in the differentiation between VT and SVT. The most commonly used criteria are those of Brugada et al. (Fig. 15.22).

Other methods of differentiating between VT and SVT, such as the Bayesian approach, and algorithms for distinguishing between VT and antidromic AVRT (which can be very challenging) may be useful in the outpatient setting, but are beyond the purview of this chapter describing acute therapies.

During the first few moments after the initiation of WCT in the CICU, a rapid assessment should be made of the patient's stability. Take note of the patient's level of consciousness, and then check the telemetry monitor.

If VF is seen on the monitor, one should expeditiously implement the published ACLS guidelines for its management. Several important practical issues should be kept in mind:

- When placing the defibrillator pads, the anteroposterior orientation is preferred.
- Management of the airway and bag-mask ventilation in anticipation of possible intubation should be performed.
- CPR should be initiated and continued whenever defibrillation or assessment of rhythm are not being performed.
- Time is of the essence; the longer a patient is in VF, the more difficult it will be to defibrillate them, and the greater the postdefibrillatory hemodynamic depression.
- The external defibrillator should be in "defibrillator" mode (monitor and pacer modes are also available) and the "sync" indicator light should be off.
- The defibrillation energy to 200 Joules (J) for a monophasic device, or 150J for a biphasic unit. Hit the charge button, and when full charge is reached (most devices emit a constant tone), indicate "all clear!" to everyone in the room. When you have verified that no team members are in contact with the patient or the bed, firmly depress the "shock"

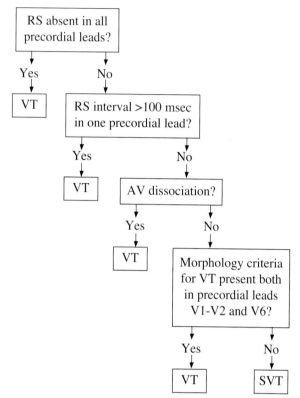

VT, ventricular tachycardia; AV, atrioventricular; SVT, supraventricular tachycardia.

FIGURE 15.22. Brugada Criteria for distinguishing ventricular tachycardia from supraventricular tachycardia with aberrant conduction, which pose four sequential questions.

button until the patient has visibly received the shock. Assess the postshock rhythm. If VF persists, shock at 300J monophasic or 200J biphasic (the maximum for these devices), then 360J monophasic (maximum) or 200J biphasic.

- If the patient has not converted to sinus or another perfusing rhythm, ACLS algorithms should be followed, depending on the rhythm encountered (pulseless electrical activity, asystole, or otherwise.)

If polymorphic VT, especially TdP, is present, one should pursue the defibrillation protocol just listed for VF, as this is also a disorganized rhythm, generally requiring high energies. Two grams of magnesium sulfate should be administered IV over 2 minutes; this simple intervention is frequently effective at converting patients from TdP.

Monomorphic VT: If the patient is pulseless or has signs of hemodynamic instability, such as acute depression of consciousness or a systolic blood pressure (SBP) <90 mmHg, the first step is to emergently cardiovert (with "sync" on), typically at 200J monophasic or 100J biphasic. In general, less energy is required for monomorphic VT, since it is a more organized, reentrant rhythm, in contrast to VF or polymorphic VT. If conversion to sinus is unsuccessful, subsequent shocks will be at 300J monophasic (150J biphasic), then at 360J monophasic (200J biphasic).

If the patient with monomorphic VT is hemodynamically stable, pharmacologic cardioversion can be attempted instead. For reasons just described, our agent of choice is amiodarone. If a single 150 mg IV bolus over 10 minutes is ineffective at breaking the VT, we will give a second bolus, followed by a 1 mg/min drip. If VT persists after two boluses of amiodarone and 20 to 30 minutes of the drip, it is then most reasonable to sedate and DC cardiovert the patient. In most cases, a full IV load of amiodarone followed by transition to oral medication will prevent further episodes of VT. However, in some cases VT will recur, necessitating addition of a second agent. Lidocaine is generally chosen, using a 1 mg/kg IV bolus over 2 minutes, which can be repeated twice, followed by a drip at 2 mg/min (usable range 1 to 4 mg/min). Since the metabolism of lidocaine is hepatic, and dependent on hepatic blood flow, patients with liver disease or heart failure should receive lower maintenance doses of lidocaine. For infusions >24 hours, levels should be monitored (therapeutic range 1.5–5 mg/mL), and the patient should be observed carefully for signs and symptoms of toxicity (drowsiness, slurred speech, paresthesias including perioral numbness, tinnitus, tremor, confusion/disorientation, seizures, and coma).

Persistent, recurrent VT is defined as VT or VF occurring two or more times in a 24-hour period, requiring multiple shocks, and is often referred to as "VT/VF storm" or "electrical storm (ES)." While this definition is conservative, and designed for research purposes, those working in the CCU often treat patients for whom the number of shocks extend well into the double digits. These episodes are often recalcitrant to one or more anti-arrhythmic medications, and are agonizing for patient and practitioner alike. Most importantly, one should seek to identify a reversible cause of the VT or VF and treat it as quickly as possible. Coronary ischemia is very likely to be driving the arrhythmia of certain patients: those with ongoing MI, with or without ST-segment elevation; those with history of MI or known CAD and symptoms suggestive of ischemia.

Nonsustained VT is usually asymptomatic, but occasionally patients complain of palpitations. NSVT can be seen in a wide variety of patients, including those with chronic CAD and cardiomyopathies (ischemic, dilated, or hypertrophic), and those with QT prolongation due to various antiarrhythmic drugs. In the CCU, most patients encountered with NSVT are those who have recently experienced an MI (45% of post-MI patients will experience NSVT within 48 hours), or are currently ischemic. As we learned from the CAST trial, suppression of postinfarction ventricular ectopy (PVCs or NSVT) with class Ic anti-arrhythmics is harmful, leading to an increase in mortality. Hence, our goal is not to treat the NSVT, but to consider reversible causes of it. In our CCU, the main concern is for the patient having ongoing ischemia leading to the NSVT. Judicious use of IV nitroglycerin and IV or oral metoprolol prior to left-heart catheterization and angiography are usually helpful in reducing ischemia, and hence, NSVT. But, in general with NSVT, it is more important to obey the maxim, "treat the patient, not the ECG."

SVT with Aberrant Conduction

Only when VT has been thoroughly excluded should one consider treating WCT as an SVT with aberrancy. As with any WCT, hemodynamic instability calls for immediate DCC.

In the hemodynamically stable patient, time may be spent to further characterize the rhythm. Review of the medical record and past ECGs may reveal previous occurrences and successfully implemented therapies. The identification of P waves can be facilitated by the use of vagal maneuvers (unilateral carotid sinus pressure) or the administration of IV adenosine (6 mg bolus, followed by 12 mg bolus if no response). Some SVTs will break with adenosine, which in these cases can serve as both diagnostic and therapeutic agent. Since the presence of a wide complex may indicate the presence of WPW, it is generally best to avoid longer-acting nodal-blocking agents such as beta blockers or calcium channel blockers. Such agents may elicit 1:1 conduction down the accessory pathway, increased ventricular rate, and hemodynamic collapse.

The most useful agent for SVT with aberrant conduction is IV procainamide, given as a 15 mg/kg bolus at 20 mg/min, followed by a 2 to 4 mg/min drip. Long-term administration of procainamide necessitates checking serum levels of the parent drug (therapeutic range 4 to 10 mg/L) and its active metabolite, N-acetylprocainamide (NAPA; <20 mg/L). For particularly challenging CCU cases and for any long-term therapy of SVT, it is reasonable to enlist the assistance of a specialist in cardiac electrophysiology (EP). Such a consultant is best equipped to manage chronic oral drug therapy or to plan a catheter-based ablation procedure.

CLINICAL PRESENTATION TIPS

- Hypotension requires immediate DCC and fluid management.
- Ischemia may be present and it is a typical cause of ventricular tachycardia. Appropriate revascularization should be performed. May benefit from IABP.
- Electrolytes: Hyperkalemia is the most common electrolyte abnormality and requires immediate therapy with calcium gluconate, insulin and D5W, and kayexalate. Hyperkalemic arrest remains the sole class I indication for the use of sodium bicarbonate.
- Mental-status change: It is typically related to hypotension and may resolve after cardioversion.
- Respiratory failure: Typically related to cerebral hypoperfusion. Requires immediate intubation to protect airway.

DISCHARGE

Patients with WCT should be kept in CICU until the underlying etiology (i.e., ischemia, electrolyte changes, medication) is corrected. Before leaving the CICU, prophylactic interventions such as ICD or ablation should be discussed and planned, together with the EP consultant. Furthermore, appropriate medications (beta blockers, calcium channel blockers) should be titrated to effective doses.

RECOMMENDED READING

1. Brugada P, Brugada J, Mont L, et al. A new approach to the differential diagnosis of a regular tachycardia with a wide QRS complex. *Circulation.* 1991; 83:1649–1659.
2. Lau EW, Pathamanathan RK, Ng GA, et al. The Bayesian approach improves the electrocardiographic diagnosis of broad complex tachycardia. *Pacing Clin Electrophysiol.* 2000; 23:1519–1526.
3. Echt DS, Liebson PR, Mitchell LB, et al. Mortality and morbidity in patients receiving encainide, flecainide, or placebo. The Cardiac Arrhythmia Suppression Trial. *N Engl J Med.* 1991; 324:781–788.

CHAPTER 16

Bradyarrhythmias

TELLY A. MEADOWS

Bradyarrhythmias are common rhythm disturbances encountered in the coronary care unit (CCU) setting and they are often caused by sinus node dysfunction or atrioventricular (AV) conduction disturbances. It is of paramount importance to diagnose the cause of the bradyarrhythmia in order to determine appropriate acute and chronic treatment strategies.

PRESENTATION

The clinical presentation of patients with bradycardia can be variable. Symptoms typically can range from fatigue or malaise to altered mental status, end-organ dysfunction, and frank shock. Symptomatic bradycardia requires immediate intervention. Asymptomatic patients may necessitate only conservative therapy (i.e., holding nodal blockers).

PHYSICAL EXAMINATION

- Arterial pulse: periodic change in amplitude in second-degree AV block; constantly changing in third-degree AV block
- Jugular venous pulse: Intermittent canon a waves in third-degree AV block
- First heart sound: softer S_1 in first-degree AV block; progressive softening S_1 in second-degree—Mobitz type I block; constantly changing S_1 in third-degree AV block
- Functional systolic ejection murmur may be heard in third-degree AV block
- Hypotension or clinical signs of shock (decreased urine output, cool or clammy extremities, or altered mental status)

ACUTE MANAGEMENT

- **Telemetry:** Determine the rhythm and monitor for pauses.

Diagnostic Tests:

- **ECG:** Determine the rhythm, rule out ischemia, and identify conduction abnormalities.
  - sinus bradycardia is a rate <60 bpm
  - sinus pauses must be longer than 3 seconds to be abnormal
  - atrioventricular block
- Autonomic Testing: Evaluate for autonomic reflexes.
  - carotid sinus massage distinguishes sinus pause from carotid hypersensitivity

Management: Review medication profile and stop any nodal blockers—beta blockers, calcium channel blockers, or digoxin.

- **Tools:** Cardiac telemetry, two large-bore IV lines, supplemental oxygen, ECG
- **Stat labs:** CMP, CBC, cardiac enzymes, TSH, digoxin level, PT, INR, PTT, pertinent drug levels/toxicology screen

Medications:

- Atropine 0.04 mg/kg IV bolus
- Dopamine 2 to 10 µg/kg/min for hypotension and bradycardia-may also consider epinephrine 2 µg/min to 10 µg/min or isoproterenol 1 µg/min
- Glucagon 3 mg followed by 3 mg/hr if necessary for beta blocker toxicity
- Digibind #vials = weight (kg) × digoxin concentration (ng/mL) ÷ 100
- Temporary transcutaneous pacing as a bridge to transvenous pacing
- Temporary transvenous pacing

Surgical: Depending on the etiology of the bradycardia, a permanent pacemaker make need to be considered.

CCU Tip: Management is dictated by symptoms related to the bradycardia. Remember to always identify and treat any reversible causes for the arrhythmia. Avoid atropine in Mobitz type II block.

DIFFERENTIAL DIAGNOSIS

Sinus Node Dysfunction
- Inappropriate sinus bradycardia
- Sinoatrial exit block
- Sinoatrial arrest
- Tachycardia-bradycardia syndrome/sick sinus syndrome

Atrioventricular Conduction Disturbances
- First-degree AV block
- Second-degree AV block: Mobitz type I or Mobitz type II
- Third-degree AV block
- Accelerated junctional rhythm

Ischemic damage to the sinoatrial and atrioventricular node is an important cause of acute bradyarrhythmia in a critical-care setting. The sinus node artery, a branch of the right coronary artery in approximately 55% to 60% of people and circumflex artery in approximately 35% to 40% of people, supplies blood to the SA node. The AV node receives its blood supply from the AV nodal artery, which arises from the posterior descending artery in approximately 80% of people, from the circumflex artery in 10%, and from both arteries in 10% of people.

Sinus nodal dysfunction (sick sinus syndrome) is the most common cause for bradyarrhythmias and may manifest clinically as inappropriate sinus bradycardia, sinus arrest, or tachycardia-bradycardia syndrome. It is also apparent in posttachycardia (i.e., atrial fibrillation) conversion pauses typically seen in the CCU setting. The most common etiology for intrinsic dysfunction of the SA node is idiopathic degenerative disease, the incidence of which increases with age. Coronary artery disease and acute myocardial ischemia are important causes for intrinsic SA nodal dysfunction. In patients with an inferior myocardial infarction, the sinus nodal dysfunction may be caused by sinus node artery ischemia or from increased vagal tone (Bezold-Jarisch reflex). Medications and excessive vagal tone as seen in vasovagal syncope and carotid hypersensitivity are the most common etiologies of extrinsic SA nodal dysfunction. Various medications including beta blockers, calcium channel blockers, digoxin, and type IA, IC, and III antiarrhythmics are known to depress the function of the SA node.

Atrioventricular conduction disturbances manifest clinically as either first-, second-, or third-degree AV block on the surface electrocardiogram. The most common causes of AV block are drugs or myocardial ischemia. Drugs can precipitate AV block either indirectly via the autonomic nervous system (beta blockers, digoxin) or through direct action on the AV node (calcium channel blockers, amiodarone). Various degrees of AV block can be seen in the setting of an acute myocardial infarction. Both inferior and anterior myocardial infarctions can result in third-degree heart block. In an acute inferior myocardial infarction, the complete heart block is usually transient and it typically occurs at the level of the AV node resulting in a junctional escape with a narrow QRS complex. In an acute anterior myocardial infarction there is a greater propensity for irreversible AV block. Anterior wall MI associated with complete heart block or a new bundle branch block or hemiblock implies a proximal LAD occlusion proximal to the first septal perforator. Thus, a proximal LAD MI is usually associated with infarction of the bundle branches with a resultant infranodal escape rhythm with a wide QRS complex. Other less frequent causes of acquired AV block include traumatic injury due to intracardiac catheterization manipulation (especially a new right bundle branch block [RBBB] in the setting of PA catheter placement) or cardiac surgery, myocarditis, infiltrative disease, and infective endocarditis especially in the presence of aortic valve involvement.

RISK FACTORS

- Age
- Prior conduction abnormalities
- Coronary artery disease (CAD) with ischemia
- Acute myocardial infarction (MI)
- Cardiac surgery
- Medications (beta blockers, digoxin, calcium channel blockers, clonidine, anti-arrhythmics)
- Excessive vagal tone, carotid sinus syndrome, vasovagal syncope
- Infiltrative cardiomyopathies (amyloidosis, sarcoidosis, hemochromatosis)
- Endocarditis
- Myocarditis (Lyme disease, Chagas' disease, tuberculosis, rheumatic fever)
- Calcific valvular disease
- Metabolic derangements (hyperkalemia, hypermagnesemia, sepsis)
- Hypothyroidism
- Hypothermia
- Obstructive sleep apnea

DIAGNOSTIC TESTS

Twelve-lead electrocardiogram is the most important diagnostic test. Proper rhythm identification, especially in AV-conduction disturbances, is vital for the management and prognosis for the patient. (Figs. 16.1 and 16.2).

Carotid sinus massage/vagal maneuvers aids in distinguishing between AV node and infranodal block in AV conduction disturbances. In carotid sinus hypersensitivity, a sinus pause/arrest may be elicited by carotid sinus massage, whereas this should not occur in intrinsic SA node disease. A positive test results in a >3 second pause and/or a 50 mmHg or greater drop in pressure. In AV conduction disturbances, a vagal maneuver will worsen an atrioventricular nodal block, but it will not typically have any affect and may actually improve an infranodal block.

Atropine administration improves conduction through the AV node and decreases AV nodal blockade. Atropine increases sinus rate, which may worsen conduction disturbances due to infranodal blockade.

Electrophysiologic testing is used to evaluate and determine the site of AV block. Sinoatrial node function is determined by the sinus-node recovery time.

MEDICAL MANAGEMENT

Initial physical exam includes assessment of end-organ hypoperfusion. Blood pressure, palpation of peripheral extremities and pulses, urine output, and assessment of mental status should be performed immediately. An evaluation of the jugular venous waveforms and pressures along with auscultation of the lungs and heart should be documented.

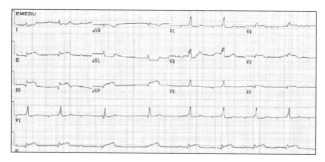

FIGURE 16.1. Inferior wall myocardial infarction with associated intermittent heart block.

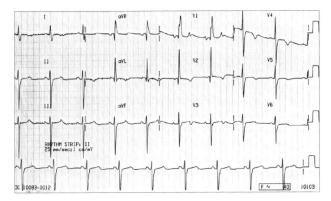

FIGURE 16.2. Second-degree atrioventricular block: Mobitz type I or Mobitz type II. An example where carotid sinus massage may be helpful to delineate the site of block.

Supplemental oxygen should be provided. All patients should be placed on cardiac telemetry with continuous pulse oximetry monitoring. A minimum of two large-bore IV sites should be established. Laboratory studies including any relevant toxicology screen or drug levels should be sent.

Asymptomatic patients with adequate systemic perfusion do not generally require any specific medical therapy or a temporary pacemaker. Cardiac monitoring and serial physical exams should be performed to ensure no decline in clinical status.

The treatment modality of choice for symptomatic bradycardia (i.e., hemodynamic compromise, ischemia, or heart failure) is pacing. Medical therapy has a limited role in its management. Acute pharmacologic therapy can serve as a bridge to temporary pacing and may allow time for the assessment and treatment of any reversible causes for the rhythm disturbance. Atropine is the immediate therapy of choice for symptomatic bradycardia. Other potential therapies include dopamine, epinephrine, glucagon (if beta-blocker overdose is suspected), and digoxin-specific Fab (if digitalis overdose suspected). Transcutaneous pacing should be considered immediately in the following patients: those with high-degree AV block (Mobitz type II second degree or third degree), those who are severely symptomatic, and those patients who do not respond to atropine. During transcutaneous pacing, palpate the pulse to ensure adequate capture as the rhythm strip can be misleading.

Identify and correct any reversible causes for the bradyarrhythmia.

CLINICAL PRESENTATION TIPS

- Fever or other signs of infection such as an elevated white blood cell count should raise suspicion of infective endocarditis, myocarditis, or Lyme disease.
- Renal failure may predispose to hyperkalemia or adverse drug effects due to lack of clearance.
- Inferior myocardial infarction associated with third-degree atrioventricular block is usually transient and may only require temporary pacing.
- Anterior myocardial infarction associated with third-degree atrioventricular block will often require permanent pacing.

COMPLICATIONS

Angina/myocardial ischemia may occur to due to bradycardia if the rate compromises coronary blood flow.

Syncope associated with bradycardia is often a presenting complaint and an ominous sign that needs to be further investigated.

Cardiogenic shock in the setting of complete heart block especially associated with acute myocardial infarction is not uncommon and must be addressed by rapid revascularization as well as temporary pacing and possibly permanent pacing.

DISCHARGE

Patients with bradyarrhythmias can be safely discharged from the intensive care unit (ICU) once the conduction disturbance has resolved or once pacing, either via a temporary transvenous (if the patient has an adequate escape in case the temporary wire is dislodged) or permanent approach, is available for those patients with an irreversible symptomatic bradyarrhythmia. Asymptomatic patients with persistent bradycardia who have been observed and do not meet any indication for permanent pacemaker placement can also be safely discharged from the ICU. While ruling out coronary artery disease is not required prior to placement of a permanent pacemaker in patients with persistent symptomatic bradycardia, stress testing should be considered at some point following permanent pacemaker placement to rule out revascularizable disease.

RECOMMENDED READING

1. Kaushik V, Leon AR, Forrester JS, et al. Bradyarrhythmias, temporary and permanent pacing. *Crit Care Med.* 2000; 28[suppl.]:N121–N128.
2. Mangrum JM, DiMarco JP. The evaluation and management of bradycardia. *N Engl J Med.* 2000; 342:703–709.
3. Gregoratos G, Abrams J, Epstein AE, et al. ACC/AHA/NASPE 2002 Guideline update for implantation of cardiac pacemakers and antiarrhythmia devices—summary article: a report of the American College of Cardiology/ American Heart Association Task Force on Practice Guidelines (ACC/ AHA/NASPE Committee to Update the 1998 Pacemaker Guidelines). *Circulation.* 2002; 106:2145–2161.
4. Wolbrette DL, Naccarelli GV. Bradycardias: sinus nodal dysfunction and atrioventricular conduction disturbances. In: Topol EJ, ed. *Textbook of Cardiovascular Medicine.* 2nd ed. Philadelphia: Lippincott Williams & Wilkins; 2002:1385–1402.

Diseases of the Aorta and Pericardium

CHAPTER 17

Acute Aortic Syndromes

THOMAS H. WANG

RYAN D. CHRISTOFFERSON

MEHDI H. SHISHEHBOR

Acute syndromes of the aorta include aortic aneurysm expansion, aortic dissection (AD), intramural hematoma (IMH), penetrating aortic ulcer (PAU) and contained aortic rupture. Aortic dissection develops from an intimal flap in the aortic wall, separating a "true" and "false" lumen. The intimal tear propagates antegrade or retrograde, causing ischemia by compromising branch vessels. Aortic dissection has an incidence of at least 2,000 cases per year in the United States, and if the dissection flap involves the ascending aorta or arch the early mortality is 1% per hour when left untreated. Any AD occurring less than 2 weeks from symptom onset is considered acute. An IMH is differentiated from AD by the finding of hematoma in the medial layer of the aorta, caused by hemorrhage within an atherosclerotic plaque or the vasa vasorum. A PAU is characterized by an ulcer in the aortic wall that penetrates beyond the intimal layer. Death occurs by aortic rupture, tamponade, or complications of malperfusion.

PRESENTATION

The typical presentation is severe tearing or stabbing chest and/or back pain that is sudden in onset. Patients with AD are often younger and have a connective tissue disorder or bicuspid aortic valve, and patients with IMH or PAU are often older with hypertension and atherosclerosis. Proximal (Type A) dissection may also present with differential upper-extremity pulses, aortic insufficiency, stroke, tamponade, or cardiac arrest. Distal (Type B) dissections present with malperfusion syndromes such as lower extremity ischemia.

ACUTE MANAGEMENT

Diagnostic Tests:

- **TTE:** Evaluate for pericardial effusion and tamponade, aortic insufficiency, aortic root dilatation, intimal flap, and wall motion.
- **CT scan (preferred):** Evaluate for AD, IMH, or PAU, define proximal and distal borders of the dissection (Type A vs. Type B), true-and-false lumen, and evaluate branch vessel involvement.
- **TEE:** Consider if patient is too ill for transport to CT or when renal impairment is present. In addition to items assessed by TTE, TEE can evaluate arch involvement, intimal flap, and flow in the true and false lumen.

Management:

- **Tools:** Arterial line, two large-bore IV lines, portable CXR
- **STAT labs:** Type and cross, CBC, CMP, PT, INR, PTT

Medications:

- IV metoprolol 5–10 mg push; may repeat every 5 minutes; until heart rate <60 and mean arterial pressure 60–65 mmHg
- Alternative: labetalol gtt 1–2 mg/min for heart rate and blood pressure control
- Nipride gtt up to 300 µg/min if heart rate reaches goal but mean arterial pressure still elevated

Surgical: Immediate surgical consultation with cardiothoracic surgery if acute Type A; vascular surgery if Type B.

CCU Tip: Pain should be controlled by adequate hemodynamic management. Opiates should be utilized when necessary.

PHYSICAL EXAMINATION

- Diastolic murmur of AI (40%–50% of Type A)
- Pulse deficit (<20% of Type A)
- Baseline neurologic exam (may have transient deficits)
- Jugular venous distention (JVD), pulsus paradoxus
- Clinical signs of hypoperfusion or shock

DIFFERENTIAL DIAGNOSIS

- Acute myocardial infarction (MI)
- Pulmonary embolus
- Aortic stenosis
- Pericarditis
- Esophageal disorders

RISK FACTORS

- Hypertension—up to 80% of patients
- Age—up to 80% of patients
- Connective tissue disease (e.g., Marfan's disease, Ehlers-Danlos syndrome)
- Family history of aneurysm
- Congenital bicuspid or unicuspid aortic valve
- Smoking
- Dyslipidemia
- Crack cocaine
- Coarctation of the aorta
- Turner's syndrome
- Giant cell arteritis
- Pregnancy
- Trauma (e.g., deceleration injury, IABP, angiography, surgery)

DIAGNOSTIC TESTS

Diagnostic imaging should be used to characterize the extent of dissection or hematoma (the beginning and endpoint), as well as branch vessel involvement. An intimal flap should be sought and antegrade, retrograde, or delayed flow into the false lumen characterized. Noncommunicating aneurysms often cannot be differentiated from IMH, which appear as a crescentic or circular thinkening of the aortic wall without Doppler-detectable flow within the wall and without intimal flap. The PAU appears as a visible crater-like outpouching of the aorta with irregular, jagged edges or associated aortic plaque. The finding of pericardial fluid or pleural fluid may be a sign of rupture in any acute aortic syndrome. Frequently, more than one imaging modality is used to diagnose AD, with CT the most common initial modality (60%).

Transthoracic echocardiography should be at the bedside immediately upon patient's arrival to the intensive care unit (ICU). It has a sensitivity of 59% to 85% and specificity of 63% to 96%. While not ideal, it is easy to obtain and can assess for aortic insufficiency, hemorrhagic pericardial effusion, and wall-motion abnormalities (to rule out myocardial infarction). In addition, normal right-ventricular (RV) function and a lack of tricuspid regurgitation make acute massive pulmonary embolus unlikely.

Computed tomography provides 83% to 94% sensitivity and 87% to 100% specificity, and should clearly define the proximal and distal edges of the dissection, as well as branch vessel involvement. It can also exclude a pericardial effusion but cannot evaluate aortic insufficiency. The proximal coronary arteries can often be visualized with CT (Figs. 17.1 and 17.2). Typically, a spiral CT protocol that includes the great vessels and the iliac arteries is needed. The need for patient transport to the CT scanner, the time required for the test, and IV contrast exposure are downsides to selection of CT as the imaging modality of choice.

Transesophageal echocardiography (TEE) has 66% to 99% sensitivity and 77% to 97% specificity for AD. Similar to transthoracic echocardiography (TTE), it can quantify aortic insufficiency, assess wall motion, and evaluate the pericardial space. In addition, it can confirm the diagnosis of Type-A dissection, when CT is contraindicated. Doppler is useful to assess flow within the true-and-false lumen, and define the intimal flap. The proximal coronary arteries are also evaluated by TEE, which can be done expeditiously at the bedside.

MRI is considered the gold standard for diagnosis with 98% sensitivity and specificity, but its use is limited acutely.

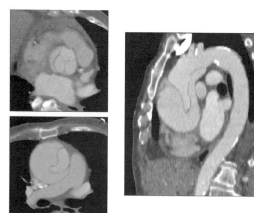

FIGURE 17.1. Type A aortic dissection demonstrated in axial and coronal CT images.

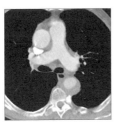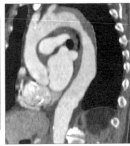

FIGURE 17.2. Type A intramural hematoma demonstrated in axial and coronal CT images.

Angiography can also be performed but like MRI, it is of limited use in the acute setting.

MEDICAL MANAGEMENT

Initial physical exam should include bilateral arm blood pressures, assessment of JVD and pulsus paradoxus. Additionally, bilateral radial pulses as well as femoral, popliteal, and dorsalis pedis pulses should be obtained. Cardiac auscultation may reveal the diastolic murmur of aortic insufficiency. This is best heard in expiration with the patient leaning forward. Presence of a diastolic murmur along the right sternal border suggests root dilatation. Finally, a baseline neurologic assessment should be documented and followed serially over time. Detailed abdominal exam and follow up is indicated. A minimum of two large-bore IV sites should be secured along with a radial arterial line and a type and screen sent with preliminary laboratory studies.

The goal in patients with acute aortic syndrome is to reduce dP/dt and thus the shear forces on the aortic lumen. Therefore, heart rate and blood-pressure control are of paramount importance. Beta blockers should be instituted with a target heart rate <60 bpm and a mean arterial pressure of 60 to 65 mmHg. IV metoprolol or IV labetolol may be used for this purpose. We use metoprolol 5 mg IV every 5 minutes until the desired heart rate is reached. Patients with acute aortic syndrome can be resistant to beta blockers due to sympathetic nervous system activation and may require repeated doses. In patients particularly resistant to beta blockers, verapamil 0.075 to 0.1 mg/kg IV over 2 minutes followed by 5 to 15 mg/hr drip may be considered.

Sodium nitroprusside should be initiated after adequate beta blockade is achieved to optimize blood pressure control. This agent should not be instituted prior to beta-blocker therapy as this may lead to reflex tachycardia and increased dP/dt.

Occasionally patients may require vasopressor therapy to maintain hemodynamic stability. The pressor of choice is either norepinephrine or phenylephrine, both of which have little effect on dP/dt. Epinephrine and dopamine should be avoided. Normal or low blood pressure mandates careful evaluation for blood loss, pericardial effusion or heart failure.

SURGICAL MANAGEMENT

Acute AD, IMH, or PAU of the ascending aorta and/or aortic arch (Type A) requires immediate surgical intervention to prevent excess mortality. In some cases, low-risk IMH and PAU in the ascending aorta and arch may be managed medically after surgical consultation. Aortic syndromes in the descending aorta (Type B) are often managed medically. However, the presence of a malperfusion syndrome, contained rupture, expanding aneurysm, intractable pain, or extension of dissection into the arch or ascending aorta constitutes an indication for surgical or interventional stent-graft management.

CLINICAL PRESENTATION TIPS

- Hypotension: suspect cardiac tamponade or ruptured dissection
- Acute MI: usually due to right coronary artery involvement
- Respiratory Distress: acute heart failure due to worsening aortic insufficiency
- Bradyarrhythmia/Heart block: extension into the right coronary artery
- Mental status change: carotid artery involvement
- Decreased Urine Output: extension of dissection into the renal arteries
- Limb ischemia: subclavian involvement for upper extremity or iliac involvement in lower extremities
- Bowel ischemia: celiac or mesenteric artery involvement
- Paraplegia: comprised flow in the anterior spinal artery

COMPLICATIONS

Pericardial effusion/tamponade is one of the most common mechanisms of death in acute proximal aortic dissection. Pericardiocentesis is **NOT** recommended as it may actually increase dP/dt and worsen the dissection. Aggressive volume resuscitation and emergent surgical intervention is necessary.

Acute MI occurs in 1% to 2% of dissection patients, and thrombolysis is contraindicated. Left-heart catheterization has high risk and low benefit in the context of acute AD.

Congestive heart failure (CHF) develops when aortic insufficiency is severe because the left ventricle is unable to dilate acutely. Diuretics are necessary and if aortic insufficiency is severe, a higher heart rate may be tolerated.

Bradyarrhythmia/heart block can be iatrogenically induced or is due to dissection involvement of the right coronary artery.

Malperfusion syndrome results from compromise of branch vessels, and leads to CVA or TIA (3% to 6% of Type-A dissections), limb ischemia, bowel infarction, renal failure, or paraplegia.

Aortic aneurysm expansion or rupture may occur in the setting of an unstable aorta with recent AD, IMH, or PAU. Risk for rupture is actually higher with IMH and PAU.

DISCHARGE

Patients with acute aortic syndromes can be safely discharged from the ICU **if surgical management is not warranted**, and the patient is pain free with adequate blood-pressure control on oral medications. The transition to oral medications should occur once decision is made for medical management. Preferred oral medications include metoprolol or labetolol for heart-rate control. Once appropriate heart rate is achieved, amlodipine and/or ACE-inhibitor may be added for tighter blood-pressure control. The dose should be titrated aggressively while simultaneously weaning off the intravenous antihypertensive agents.

RECOMMENDED READING

1. Mukherjee D, Eagle KA. Aortic dissection—an update. *Curr Probl Cardiol.* 2005; 30:287–325.
2. Nienaber CA, Eagle KA. Aortic dissection: new frontiers in diagnosis and management: Part II: therapeutic management and follow-up. *Circulation.* 2003; 108:772–778.
3. Nienaber CA, Eagle KA. Aortic dissection: new frontiers in diagnosis and management: Part I: from etiology to diagnostic strategies. *Circulation.* 2003; 108:628–635.
4. Lissin LW, Vagelos R. Acute aortic syndrome: a case presentation and review of the literature. *Vasc Med.* 2002; 7:281–287.

CHAPTER 18

Pericardial Tamponade

SAIF ANWARUDDIN

Pericardial tamponade occurs due to fluid accumulation in the pericardial space, causing hemodynamic compromise by impairing diastolic filling of the atria and ventricles. The most crucial determinants for the development of tamponade are the rate of fluid accumulation and the compliance of the pericardium. Whereas large amounts of fluid that slowly accumulate may not lead to tamponade physiology, smaller amounts of fluid can lead to tamponade if accumulation occurs rapidly. The pericardial space typically holds 15 to 30 cc of fluid and can take on approximately 200 cc of fluid in a rapid fashion before significant changes are noted. Loculated pericardial effusions also can cause tamponade by way of localized compression of either atria or ventricles and are commonly encountered postoperatively.

Rapid fluid accumulation in the pericardium impairs diastolic filling of the heart. Compromise of the right atrium typically occurs first as it is the lowest pressure chamber. This is followed by diastolic collapse of the right ventricle as the pressure in the pericardial space exceeds the diastolic pressure within the right ventricle. The degree of diastolic filling impairment may be transient; restricted to early diastole or may progress to involve the entire filling period. Consequently, there is inappropriate filling of the right atrium and right ventricle, leading to an increase in central venous pressures characterized by raised jugular venous pressure (JVP) on exam and a plethoric inferior vena cava (IVC) that fails to collapse on inspiration on echo.

PRESENTATION

The presenting symptoms of cardiac tamponade are quite nonspecific, and, thus, a high degree of suspicion must be maintained in the appropriate

A C U T E M A N A G E M E N T

Diagnostic Tests:

- **TTE (preferred):** Evaluate for effusion, size, presence of dissection flap, systolic collapse of right atrium, right ventricle or left atrium, respiratory variation across the mitral and triscupid valves, inferior vena cava plethora.
  - Respiratory variation is defined as >25% decreased flow across the mitral valve or >40% decreased flow across the tricuspid valve with inspiration (measured by continuous wave Doppler.
  - Inferior vena cava plethora with failure to decrease by 50% in size upon deep inspiration
- **CXR:** May show recently enlarged cardiac silhouette without evidence of pulmonary edema
- **ECG:** In the setting of a large pericardial effusion, ECG may demonstrate low voltages and electrical alternans (Fig. 18.1)
- **TEE:** Especially helpful in post-operative patients when assessing for loculated effusions causing tamponade physiology.
- **RHC:** To assess for equalization of pressures and response to therapy. Will also be needed for suspected superimposed constrictive physiology during pericardiocentesis.

Management:

- **Tools:** Two large-bore IVs and/or central venous access, transthoracic echocardiography, pericardiocentesis kit.
- **STAT Labs:** Type and Cross, CBC, CMP, PT, INR, PTT

Medications:

- IV normal saline wide open
- Blood products to maintain a hemoglobin of ~10 mg/dL
- Consider, IV dopamine if hypotensive despite fluid resuscitation
- Discontinue all anticoagulation

Surgical: Consider surgical consultation if the effusion is located posteriorly or if there is a complication with the pericardiocentesis.

CCU Tip: Tamponade is a clinical diagnosis and patients quickly deteriorate. Fluids, pressors, and pericardiocentesis should be performed immediately and without delay.

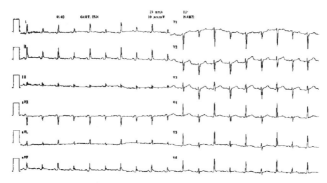

FIGURE 18.1. ECG demonstrating electrical alternans as well as low voltage.

clinical situation. Often patients are lethargic and appear quite ill. Respiratory effort is often increased and patients can appear diaphoretic; with evidence of cool and clammy peripheries. An accurate history, especially for recent percutaneous procedures or open-heart surgery is necessary. Uremia and a history of malignancy should be considered. In endemic areas and in immunosupressed individuals tuberculosis should be considered.

PHYSICAL EXAMINATION

- Systemic hypotension with evidence of hypoperfusion
- Tachycardia (although bradycardia can be present in certain situations, including hypothyroidism)
- Elevated JVP (unless patient is hypovolemic) with exaggerated × descent.
- Tachypnea
- Muffled heart sounds (with large effusions)
- On auscultation, there may be egophony at the left base from large effusions
- Pericardial rub (especially when inflammatory effusions are present)
- Pulsus paradoxus—Pulsus paradoxus is noted to be an inspiratory decline in systolic blood pressure by >10 mmHg. This process is not specific to tamponade and can be seen in severe obstructive lung disease, right-ventricular (RV) infarction, large bilateral pleural effusions and following a large pulmonary embolus. Of note, pulsus paradoxus may be absent in those with severe left-ventricular (LV) dysfunction, atrial septal defects, RV hypertrophy, severe diastolic dysfunction, and loculated/localized effusions.

DIFFERENTIAL DIAGNOSIS

- Hypovolemic shock
- Constrictive pericarditis
- Acute aortic dissection extending into pericardium leading to tamponade
- RV infarction
- Pulmonary embolism

RISK FACTORS

- Malignancy
- Trauma to chest wall or upper abdomen
- Connective tissue disease
- Recent cardiac interventions
- Recent open-heart surgery
- Infection
- Renal failure (uremia)
- Aortic dissection
- Drugs
- Anticoagulation
- Indwelling catheters

DIAGNOSTIC TESTS

Transthoracic echocardiography (TTE) assesses the presence, size, and location of an effusion and any hemodynamic derangements. Echocardiographic examination can identify:

- Right-atrial systolic collapse: Elevated intracardiac pressures can cause collapse of the thin-walled right atrium. It is a very sensitive but nonspecific sign of tamponade. The longer the right-atrial collapse persists, the more specific it is for tamponade.
- RV diastolic collapse: RV diastolic collapse occurs when intrapericardial pressure exceeds RV diastolic pressure. This is a sensitive and very specific finding in tamponade. Elevated right-sided pressures in the setting of RV hypertrophy or pulmonary hypertension can prevent diastolic collapse (Fig. 18.2).
- Respiratory variation in atrioventricular flow: The respiratory cycle affects intracardiac filling and hemodynamics in an otherwise healthy individual, and this effect is exaggerated in cardiac tamponade. Inspi-

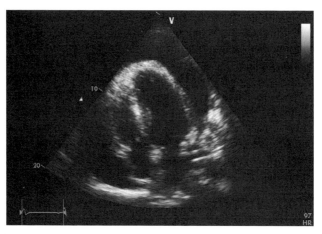

FIGURE 18.2. Circumferential effusion with right-ventricular and right-atrial collapse.

ration can decrease flow between the left atrium and left ventricle and increase flow across the tricuspid valve. By pulsed-wave Doppler echocardiographic examination, variations in flow across both the tricuspid and mitral valves can be assessed. A decrease of >25% in the flow across the mitral valve (E wave) or >40% across the tricuspid valve (E wave) is highly suspicious for tamponade.

- Respiratory variation in ventricular filling: This echocardiographic finding correlates with the clinical finding of cardiac tamponade. On echocardiography, inspiratory increase in RV volume occurs with decrease of LV volume, with movement of the septum into the LV cavity during inspiration.
- Plethora of the IVC: During deep inspiration, failure of the dilated (>2.5 cm in diameter) IVC to collapse by at least 50% of its diameter is a sensitive marker for the presence of cardiac tamponade (Fig. 18.3).

Right-heart catheterization, while not typically used as a primary diagnostic modality in cardiac tamponade, can yield important diagnostic information regarding intracardiac hemodynamics. Furthermore, it can be used to assess the success of pericardiocentesis.

- Equalization of pressures of the right atrium, the RV diastolic pressure, the pulmonary arterial diastolic pressure and the pulmonary capillary wedge pressure is the hallmark of pericardial tamponade (Fig. 18.4). It is believed that this finding is the result of a constant pericardial pressure exerting its effect on all chambers of the heart.

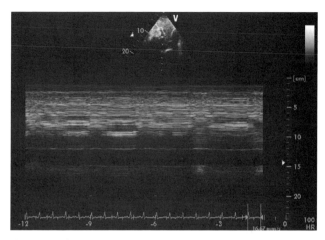

FIGURE 18.3. IVC plethora—no collapse on inspiration.

- Pressure tracing of the right atrium reveal no changes in the A or V wave of the right-heart tracing. Instead, what is observed is the absence of the y descent following the V wave.

  Transesophageal echocardiography (TEE) is limited to specific settings (in the setting of tamponade).

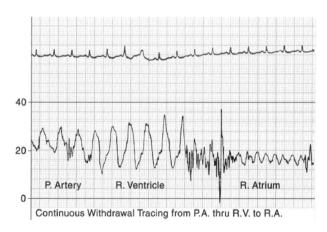

FIGURE 18.4. RHC tracing showing diastolic equalization of pressures in tamponade.

- When TTE is not sufficient in providing adequate pictures regarding the location of the fluid.
- Postoperative patients where a loculated effusion or hematoma may need to be visualized prior to surgical intervention.

Arterial line, while not required for the diagnosis of cardiac tamponade, can be helpful in establishing the diagnosis and in monitoring response to therapy. On an arterial line, it is easy to visualize pulsus paradoxus. In fact, after drainage of pericardial fluid, the loss of the exaggerated drop in blood pressure and increase in systolic blood pressure are usually observed.

MEDICAL MANAGEMENT

The initial physical exam should include assessment of jugular venous distention (JVD), pulsus paradoxus, and blood pressure. Diminished heart sounds, tachycardia, and tachypnea should also be assessed. Tamponade is a clinical diagnosis based on these features and an echo should be obtained quickly to confirm the diagnosis.

Fluid resuscitation via two large-bore IV sites should be rapidly instituted with a type and screen and coagulation panel sent for consideration of pericardiocentesis.

Maintenance of hemodynamic stability and prompt drainage are the cornerstone of acute management.

The approach to drain the fluid percutaneously or surgically depends on a number of factors.

Pericardial fluid obtained should be send for cell count, cultures, and cytology to determine etiology (i.e., malignant effusion) and initiate appropriate long-term treatment (i.e., chemotherapy, antibiotics, etc.).

SURGICAL MANAGEMENT

The size and location of the effusion, whether the collection is loculated or a result of an open-heart operative procedure, physician preferences, and hemodynamic instability are important factors to consider. Typically, large anterior, lateral, and apical pericardial effusions can be drained via a percutaneous approach using echocardiographic guidance. Surgical drainage is preferred for loculated effusions, hematomas, and for postoperative patients.

CLINICAL PRESENTATION TIPS

- Beck's Triad: Hypotension, tachycardia, diminished heart sounds
- Dyspnea: due to compressive atelectasis, elevated pulmonary arterial pressures
- Low output symptoms: Decreased mental status, low urine output, fatigue
- Dysphagia: may be due to esophageal compression

DISCHARGE

Patients with cardiac tamponade may be safely discharged from the ICU after a pericardiocentesis and/or a pericardial drain has been placed. Care must be taken in patients with malignancy-induced tamponade that the fluid does not recur. If a drain is placed, typically <50 cc/day of fluid indicates that the drain can be discontinued. Typically, these should not be left in place longer than 24 hours due to infection risks. A follow-up echocardiogram immediately after pericardiocentesis and the following morning should be performed. A CXR immediately after to rule out a pneumothorax is mandatory. A follow up CXR 12 to 24 hours later should be performed as a trivial leak may be missed on initial evaluation.

RECOMMENDED READING

1. Topol EJ. *Textbook of Cardiovascular Medicine.* 2nd ed. Lippincott Williams & Wilkins, 2002.
2. Griffin BP, Topol EJ. *Manual of Cardiovascular Medicine.* 2nd ed. Lippincott Williams & Wilkins, 2004.
3. Spodick DH. Acute cardiac tamponade. *N Engl J Med.* 2003; 349:684–690.

CHAPTER 19

Constrictive Pericarditis

THOMAS H. WANG

Constrictive pericarditis is due pericardial thickening and fibrosis often with calcification. Systolic function is unimpaired, but diastolic filling is hindered by the pericardium. Right- and left-heart failure develops as a result of decreased diastolic filling.

PRESENTATION

Constrictive pericarditis generally begins with vague symptoms that gradually progress from fatigue and malaise to dyspnea, orthopnea, and paroxysmal nocturnal dyspnea. As it progresses, right-heart failure symptoms predominate with development of peripheral edema and ascites. ECG often reveals low voltage and flattened T waves as well as left-atrial enlargement. Atrial fibrillation often occurs in conjunction with constriction.

PHYSICAL EXAMINATION

- Sinus tachycardia—chronic or subacute constriction is often seen with atrial fibrillation
- Jugular venous distention (JVD) with Kussmaul's sign (an inspiratory increase in JVD)
- Jugular venous pressure (JVP) with rapid y descent (secondary to rapid ventricular filling in early diastole)
- Decreased heart sounds, soft S_1, pericardial knock in diastole (the pericardial knock can be emphasized by squatting, sitting up, or standing)

ACUTE MANAGEMENT

Diagnostic Tests:

- **TTE:** Evaluate for septal "bounce" during diastole, IVC plethora, and impaired left ventricular filling during inspiration
  - check for decreased mitral flow and increased tricuspid flow during inspiration
  - increased systolic and diastolic pulmonary venous flow during expiration
  - pericardial thickening or calcification
  - flattening of the left-ventricular free wall
  - premature opening of the pulmonary valve
  - septal bowing toward the right ventricle during systole
- **CT scan/MRI:** Evaluate for pericardial thickening and calcification
- **TEE:** May be used to supplement/confirm TTE findings but rarely necessary
- **Right Heart Catheterization:** Equalization (<5 mmHg) of diastolic pressures.
  - Right-atrial pressure: w-shaped morphology. Prominent A wave and sharp x and y descents
  - left-ventricular and right-ventricular pressures: dip and plateau shape—"square root sign"—ventricular interdependence can be seen with simultaneous left-ventricular and right-ventricular pressures with decreased left-ventricular pressures and increased right-ventricular pressures during inspiration.

Management:

- **Tools:** Swan-Ganz catheter to guide fluid management
- **STAT labs:** CBC, CMP, PT, INR, PTT, type, and screen

Medications:

- Optimize fluid status with diuresis and low-sodium diet
- Start a beta blocker once fluid status is optimized to prevent atrial fibrillation and to augment diastolic filling

Surgical: Immediate surgical consultation if the patient is severely decompensated for pericardiectomy

CCU Tip: Consider it in patients with heart failure and normal EF. The most rapid way of diagnosing constriction is typically via a Swan-Ganz catheter showing equalization of pressures and an echocardiogram confirming the hemodynamic findings. Respiratory variation and ventricular interdependence should be confirmed.

- RV failure: ascites, peripheral edema, hepatomegaly, splenomegaly out of proportion with left-ventricular (LV) failure
- Pulsus paradoxus (inspiratory decline in systolic blood pressure greater than 10 mmHg) with effusive constriction

DIFFERENTIAL DIAGNOSIS

- Restrictive cardiomyopathy
- Diastolic heart failure
- Right-atrial tumors (myxoma)
- SVC syndrome
- Nephrotic syndrome

RISK FACTORS

- Postmyocardial infarction
- Postcardiac surgery
- Post-ICD/PPM or epicardial lead placement
- Radiation therapy
- Uremia
- Infection-viral, tuberculosis, fungal, parasitic
- Inflammatory-rheumatoid arthritis, lupus, scleroderma, sarcoid
- Trauma-blunt, penetrating, or postesophageal varices sclerotherapy
- Drugs-procainamide, methysergide, hydralazine
- Amyloid, Asbestosis, Hypereosinophilic syndromes
- Cancer

DIAGNOSTIC TESTS

Chest x-ray will predominately reveal calcification. Additionally, a dilated superior vena cava and azygos vein can often be seen.

Transthoracic echocardiography (TEE) can be utilized to detect constriction via a variety of signs:

- Respiratory variation across the mitral and tricuspid valves (Fig. 19.1). Typically, a decrease of >25% across the mitral valve and an increase of >40% across the tricuspid valve during inspiration is indicative of significant respiratory variation.
- A septal bounce may be seen during diastole; during diastole, there may be anterior movement of the septum into the RV (Fig. 19.2).
- Inferior vena cava plethora due to elevated right-sided pressures.
- Pericardial thickening or brightening of the pericardium.

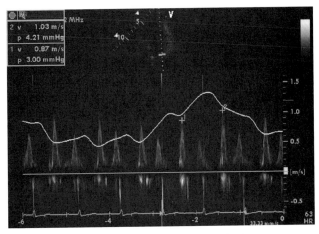

FIGURE 19.1. Respiratory variation across the mitral valve.

- Pulmonary venous flow shows increased systolic and diastolic flow during expiration. (Fig. 19.3). This helps to distinguish constriction from restriction, since there are no respiratory variations in restrictive pericarditis (Fig. 19.4).
- The LV free wall may appear flattened due to the pericardial constraint on the chamber.

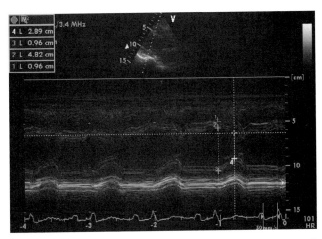

FIGURE 19.2. M-mode through the left-ventricular documenting a diastolic bounce.

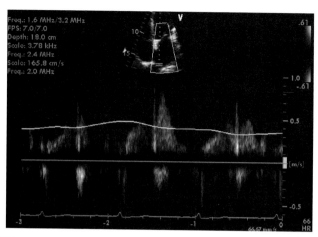

FIGURE 19.3. Pulmonary venous waveform with increased systolic and diastolic flow in expiration.

- The pulmonary valve can open early due to RV end-diastolic pressure exceeding the pulmonary arterial pressure.

Computed tomography/MRI demonstrates enlarged vena cava and left-atrial enlargement. The ventricular septum can be bowed as well. The pericardium is rarely more than 15 mm thick and calcification can be well visualized. These imaging modalities provide guidance for surgical therapy and approach.

Right- and left-heart catheterization reveals near equalization of diastolic pressures. Thus, the pulmonary capillary wedge pressure will

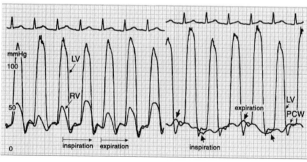

FIGURE 19.4. Ventricular interdependence and respiratory variation are seen in this example.

equal the right atrial pressure, the pulmonary artery diastolic pressure, and the RV diastolic pressure. Both the LV and the RV traces have a dip and plateau sign (the square-root sign).Right-atrial pressure tracings show characteristic x and y descents with the y descent greater than the x descent. Simultaneous LV and RV pressures will reveal equalized pressures with a decreased left ventricular end diastolic pressure (LVEDP).

MEDICAL MANAGEMENT

Medical management does not definitively address constriction unless there is an inflammatory component. To prevent fluid overload, a low-sodium diet and diuresis is recommended. A Swan-Ganz catheter is useful to help optimize the patient's volume status and care must be taken to prevent over diuresis.

Prevention of atrial fibrillation is paramount as a rapid heart rate decreases diastolic filling time and prevents adequate cardiac output. Once the fluid status is addressed, beta blockade may be considered to decrease heart rate and increase diastolic filling while also providing prophylaxis against atrial arrhythmias.

Anti-inflammatory agents such as an NSAID could be considered but are generally of minimal benefit and corticosteroids typically fail to prevent constriction after it has been surgically treated.

SURGICAL MANAGEMENT

Pericardiectomy is the treatment of choice and typically provides improvement for the majority of patients. There is an operative mortality of 5% to 20%, so patients' selection is critical.

CLINICAL PRESENTATION TIPS

- Hypotension can be due to overdiuresis or an overtly rapid heart rate limiting diastolic filling.
- Atrial fibrillation and arrhythmias are common in aggressive subacute constriction.
- Congestive heart failure (CHF) may be due to inadequate diuresis.
- Ischemia may be present since constrictive pericarditis and coronary artery disease (CAD) share some of the same risk factors (i.e., radiation).

Atypical Constriction

Local constriction may not always be generalized to the LV, but instead may be localized to the atrium, the RV, or the vena cava.

Effusive constriction is similar to pericardial tamponade in that there is a pulsus paradoxicus (lacking in pure constriction) with a large x descent in pulmonary catheter wave forms. However, Kussmaul's sign is common in this variant, and there is a lack of a rapid-filling period which distinguishes it from tamponade.

Elastic constriction can be due to a malignancy or blood deposition in the pericardium causing a clinical presentation similar to tamponade.

Transient constriction can occur in association with acute pericarditis.

DISCHARGE

Patients with acute decompensated heart failure due to contrictive pericardial disease can typically be safely discharged after the patient's volume status and atrial arrhythmias are addressed. Patients should be on an adequate diet, diuretic, and rate-controlling agent such as metoprolol, prior to discharge.

RECOMMENDED READING

1. Klein, et al. Differentiation of constrictive pericarditis from restrictive cardiomyopathy by Doppler transesophageal echocardiographic measurements of respiratory variations in pulmonary venous flows. *J Am Coll Cardiol.* 1993; 22:1935–1943.
2. Fowler, N. Constrictive pericarditis: its history and current status. *Clin Cardiol.* 1995; 18:341–350.
3. Hatle LK, et al. Differentiation of constrictive pericarditis and restrictive cardiomyopathy by Doppler echocardiography. *Circulation.* 1989; 79:357–370.

Acute Decompensated Heart Failure

CHAPTER 20

Ischemic and Nonischemic Cardiomyopathy

RYAN P. DALY

eart failure (HF) is a complex clinical syndrome characterized by impairment of the heart's ability to meet the body's circulatory needs. Ischemic cardiomyopathy occurs in patients with severe coronary disease who have had a prior myocardial infarction (MI), or have evidence of hibernating myocardium. The presence of coronary artery disease alone does not equate with ischemic cardiomyopathy, the ventricular dysfunction and wall motion abnormalities should be congruent with coronary artery stenoses and location of past infarctions. Nonischemic cardiomyopathy or dilated cardiomyopathy is also a common cause of heart failure of which familial cardiomyopathy represents 30% of these cases.

PRESENTATION

Heart failure is a clinical syndrome and must be diagnosed by careful history and physical. Therefore, patients with heart failure can present in a variety of ways. Acute pulmonary edema is the most dramatic and is characterized by the onset of dyspnea that can progress to respiratory failure. Another presentation is volume overload, with shortness of breath, orthopnea, nighttime cough and nocturia, lower extremity or dependent (if nonambulatory) edema, increasing abdominal girth, and sometimes abdominal pain and anorexia (suggestive of right-heart failure and hepatic congestion). In advanced cases, there may be paroxysmal nocturnal dyspnea (PND). Patients are commonly classified clinically by their New York Heart Association (NYHA) functional class (I–IV).

ACUTE MANAGEMENT

Diagnostic Tests:

- **History and Physical:** Evaluate for precipitating factors including a social history, travel history and family history. Check for physical exam findings of heart failure.
- **ECG:** There is no specific finding for cardiac heart failure, but the ECG will give clues to diagnosis (i.e., acute infarction, chamber enlargement or hypertrophy, etc...).
- **CXR:** Evaluate for cephalization, Kerley B lines, perihilar infiltrates, pleural effusions, and an enlarged cardiac silhouette.
- **TTE:** Evaluate for wall motion abnormalities, systolic function, diastolic dysfunction, valvular heart disease, or mechanical complications postinfarction.
- **PA catheter:** A Swan-Ganz catheter may assist in defining cardiogenic versus noncardiogenic shock and can provide short-term hemodynamically guided therapy with diuretics, vasodilators, and possibly inotropes.
- **LHC:** consider a heart catheterization with possible intervention in patients with suspected ischemia.

Management

- Telemetry, two large-bore IVs, high-flow oxygen, assess rhythm, PA catheter
- **STAT Labs:** CBC, CMP, BNP, INR, PTT, type and screen, cardiac enzymes, ABG (frequently respiratory alkalosis).
- **Diuretics:** IV lasix as needed.
- **Vasodilators:**
  - Nitrates are useful in ischemic patients and may be given sublingually 0.4–0.8 mg, as needed initially.
  - Intravenous nitrates may be started at 20 µg/kg/min to be titrated as necessary.
  - Nitroprusside may be added after nitrates have been implemented in ischemic patients or without nitrates in nonischemic patients starting with 0.2 µg/kg/min and can be aggressively titrated as necessary with a goal MAP of 65 to 70.
- **Inotropes:**
  - Dobutamine may be considered in severely compromised patients starting at 2.5 to 5 µg/kg/min. Watch for atrial or ventricular tachyarrhythmias.

- Milrinone may be utilized started with a slow IV bolus of 50 µg/kg followed by an infusion of 0.375 to 0.750 µg/kg/min for up to 48 hours.
- **Vasopressors:** Consider norepinephrine and/or dopamine in severe hypotension.
- **IABP:** Utilize in patients in cardiogenic shock if vasodilators cannot be implemented due to hypotension if there are no contraindications (aortic insufficiency, PVD, or aortic pathology.

Surgical: Consider surgical support in the setting of maximal medical therapy with an IABP for possible LVAD support and consideration for transplantation.

CCU Tip: Aggressive afterload reduction of patients in heart failure will often improve urine output and prevent acute pulmonary edema.

Evaluation of the patient before action is critical to avoid disastrous mistakes like giving nitrates in critical aortic stenosis or diuresing someone in tamponade.

Hyponatremia is an indicator of advanced heart failure.

PHYSICAL EXAMINATION

- Vitals: Tachycardia, tachypnea, hypoxia narrow pulse pressure, and hypotension may be present.
- Altered mental status, pallor, diaphoresis, frothy pink sputum. Labored breathing (Cheynes-Stokes Respirations) and anxiety.
- Cardiac: Elevated jugular venous pressure (JVP), tachycardia, murmur of valvular stenosis or regurgitation, +S3, +S4, PMI may be large (>3 cm) and laterally displaced.
- Lungs: Rales or even wheezes (cardiac asthma).
- Abdomen: Evaluation for ascites, hepatomegaly, or pulsatile liver.
- Extremities: Peripheral edema, cool and clammy skin.

DIFFERENTIAL DIAGNOSIS

Systolic Failure
- Ischemia, valvular, infectious, peripartum failure, thiamine deficiency, thyrotoxicosis, toxin mediated, idiopathic.

Diastolic Failure
- Ischemia, hypertrophic cardiomyopathy, restriction (sarcoid, amyloid, Fabry's, hemochromatosis).

Noncardiogenic Pulmonary Edema
- ARDS, re-expansion pulmonary edema, high-altitude pulmonary edema, neurogenic pulmonary edema, transfusion related acute lung injury (TRALI), opiate-induced pulmonary edema, salicylate overdose.

Miscellaneous
- Pulmonary embolism, pneumothorax, pneumonia.

PRECIPITATING FACTORS

Precipitating factors for heart failure include dietary and medicine non-compliance, ischemia, occult infection (pneumonia or UTI), toxins (EtOH or NSAIDs), endocrine disorders (hyper- or hypothyroidism), hypertension, and acute valvular dysfunction.

DIAGNOSTIC TESTS

A detailed **history and physical examination** are key to accurate diagnoses and appropriate management. Evaluate for risk factors including a social and family history.

ECG is useful to evaluate for myocardial ischemia, inappropriate brady- or tachyarrhythmias, chamber enlargement, and low voltage (infiltrative diseases or effusion).

CXR evaluates for cardiomegaly, cephalization, Kerley B lines, and perihilar infiltrates. Bilateral pleural effusions may also occur. *A clear CXR does not rule out severe LV dysfunction or pulmonary edema.*

Laboratory tests, in addition to the basic laboratory panel, include a TSH and, ferritin, fasting iron/TIBC to assess for hemochromatosis. Also, screen for HIV if the clinical suspicion is high. Check titers for Chagas antibodies in people who have traveled to endemic areas. Viral titers are not routinely checked in suspected viral myocarditis. Brain natriuretic peptide (BNP) can be helpful if there is doubt regarding the diagnosis. Finally, cardiac enzymes need to be checked to rule out an ischemic etiology. Additionally hyponatremia, transaminasemia, and pre-renal azotemia are signs of severe heart failure. Consider using the fractional excretion of urea to assess kidney status in patients with heart failure who have received diuretics.

TTE allows for assessing LV function, structural, and wall-motion abnormalities. Pay close attention to possible valve, pericardial, or RV abnormalities. All valves should be interrogated for stenotic or regurgitant lesions. Assess the diastolic function (restrictive or constrictive physiology) and check for LVOT obstructive physiology.

RHC allows for accurate assessment of hemodynamics and tailored therapy. It may be useful in a suspected mechanical complication of MI (VSD, papillary muscle rupture, or free-wall rupture) and provides important information about filling pressures allowing one to distinguish between cardiogenic and noncardiogenic shock and between cardiogenic and (noncardiogenic) pulmonary edema. Useful in assisting short-term titration of diuretics, vasodilator therapy, inotropes.

LHC is useful for patients presenting with heart failure (HF) who have chest pain and who have not had evaluation of their coronary anatomy, and is helpful in identifying ischemia as a cause of decompensation.

PET/MRI detects ischemia and viability in patient if necessary.

MEDICAL MANAGEMENT

In the acute setting, medical therapy should be focused on optimizing the patient's fluid status. To prevent fluid overload, diuresis should be considered with a low-sodium diet, and a Swan-Ganz cather can be considered for hemodynamic guidance.

In patients with adequate blood pressure reduction of preload and afterload through vasodilation is a mainstay in the treatment of acute cardiogenic pulmonary edema. **Nitrates** are useful in patients with ischemia as it rapidly reduces preload. It can be given sublingually 0.4–0.8 mg every 5 minutes as needed while an intravenous line is prepared. It can then be infused starting at 10 µg/min and uptitrated as necessary. It should be avoided in patients with aortic stenosis. **Nitroprusside** is potent vasodilator with rapid onset and can be started at 0.2 µg/kg/min and uptitrated with a goal mean arterial pressure of 65 mmHg. In an ischemic patient, IV nitroglycerin should be given prior to nitroprusside to prevent coronary steal. Cyanide toxicity is very rare and can manifest as delirium, abdominal pain, lactic acidosis, and seizures. Treat toxicity with amyl nitrate and/or sodium thiosulfate 12.5 gm in 50 mL of 5% D5W over 10 minutes. Consider dialysis if the toxicity is severe.

Inotropes may be given to provide hemodynamic support in the acutely ill patient in cardiogenic shock. **Milrinone** may be given with a slow IV bolus of 50 µg/kg followed by an infusion of 0.375 to 0.75 µg/kg/min. It can be considered in patients not responsive to dobutamine or given in addition to dobutamine. It is contraindicated in severe aortic stenosis, hypertrophic cardiomyopathy, and acute myocardial infarction. **Dobutamine** may be given at 2.5 μg/kg/min and uptitrated as necessary but may worsen tachyarrhythmias and hypotension. Avoid the use of morphine, NSAIDs, and non-dihydropyridine calcium channel blockers in patients with heart failure.

Vasopressors may be necessary in the setting of severe hypotension and so norepinephrine and/or dopamine may be implemented as necessary.

Mechanical support with an intra-aortic balloon pump or ventricular assist device may be considered in severe HF. Please refer to the mechanical circulatory support chapter.

SURGICAL MANAGEMENT

In ischemic cardiomyopathy, consider revascularization in the setting of left main or multivessel coronary disease not amenable to percutaneous coronary intervention. For nonischemic cardiomyopathy, consider mechanical support and/or transplantation if the patient is a candidate (Chapter 24).

COMPLICATIONS

Renal failure: Overdiuresis and artificially lowering mean arterial pressure (MAP) to below renal perfusion pressure can lead to decrease urine output and renal insufficiency. Many medications used in HF can worsen renal function.

Infection: This is a major cause of morbidity and mortality in the HF population. Maintain sterile technique at all times. Work up fevers and other signs of infection.

Medication side effects: Monitor patients for hyperkalemia and hypotension.

ICD Evaluation: Refer appropriate patients for internal cardiac defibrillator (ICD) placement or biventricular cardiac resynchronization therapy (BIV CRT).

DISCHARGE

Patients may be discharged from the ICU after they are hemodynamically stable and off intravenous vasodilator or vasopressor therapy. Typically, patients are transitioned off afterload therapy with a short acting ACE inhibitor such as captopril 6.25 mg three times daily, which is rapidly uptitrated. In the setting of renal insufficiency, hydralazine and isordil may be considered. Diuretics should be titrated and spironolac-tone or eplerenone may be considered. Additionally, a beta blocker such as carvedilol 6.25 mg twice daily should be implemented if possible. Patients need to be educated regarding their dietary restrictions, moni-toring of weight, and risk-factor modification.

RECOMMENDED READING

1. Ware L, et al. Acute pulmonary edema. *N Engl J Med* 2005; 353:2788–2796.
2. Sharkey, S. *A Guide to Interpretation of Hemodynamic Data in the Coronary Care Unit*. Lippincott Williams & Wilkins, 1997.
3. Hunt S, et al. ACC/AHA 2005 guideline update for the diagnosis and man-agement of chronic heart failure in the adult. *J Am Coll of Cardiol.* 2005; 46:1116–1143.
4. Wagoner et al. Cardiac function and heart failure. *J Am Coll Cardiol.* 2006; 37(11 supp):D18–D22.

CHAPTER 21

Right-Ventricular Failure

YULI Y. KIM

R ight-ventricular (RV) failure is a clinical syndrome that results from a variety of disease states. It can present as an entity isolated to the RV or, more commonly, it is associated with left-ventricular (LV) failure. In the acute setting, it is helpful to group the etiologies of RV failure as secondary to pressure overload, volume overload, or decreased contractility. Some disease entities encompass more than one process. It is important to determine the acuity of right-heart dysfunction as the pathophysiology and clinical presentation will differ.

The term *cor pulmonale* refers to RV dysfunction as a result of pulmonary hypertension from pulmonary disease or pulmonary vascular disease. Examples include pulmonary embolus, chronic obstructive pulmonary disease (COPD), and primary pulmonary hypertension. Pulmonary hypertension is discussed in further detail in Chapter 22. RV infarction is another cause of RV failure that is discussed in Chapter 5.

PRESENTATION

The presenting symptoms of RV failure depend on the underlying cause and can include fatigue, dyspnea, presyncope, or syncope. Pulmonary emboli, RV infarction, or severe pulmonary hypertension can present with chest pain. If there is underlying chronic RV dysfunction, patients can present with tender hepatomegaly, lower-extremity edema, and less commonly ascites. Massive or submassive pulmonary embolism can present as cardiac arrest.

A C U T E   M A N A G E M E N T

Diagnostic Tests:

- **TTE:** Evaluate for right-ventricular failure, left-ventricular failure, pericardial disease. Look for valvular disease as well as shunt across interatrial or ventricular septum. Obtain TEE if poor windows.
- **CT scan:** Look for central pulmonary embolus, parenchymal lung disease, pulmonary edema.
- **V/Q scan:** Assess for pulmonary embolus.
- **Cardiac MR:** Useful for evaluating congenital heart disease, right-ventricular cardiomyopathy (e.g., arrhythmogenic RV dysplasia), pericardial disease.

Management:

- **Tools:** ECG, CXR, IV access, arterial line
- **STAT labs:** CBC with differential, CMP, PT/INR, PTT, CK, CK-MB, Troponin, BNP, D-dimer, ABG
- Pulmonary artery (PA) catheterization to guide therapy
- IV fluids, pressors, inotropes
- Intra-aortic balloon pump (IABP) if cardiac index is low despite the above
- Right-ventricular infarction—immediate revascularization with percutaneous coronary intervention (PCI) indicated

Surgical: Obtain surgical consult for those patients in whom RVAD could be a potential bridge to transplant or to destination therapy. Patients in whom ECMO is considered should have surgical consults early in the hospital course. Patients with pulmonary embolus who are hemodynamically unstable and have contraindications to thrombolysis should be referred immediately for surgical embolectomy.

CCU Tip: In mechanically ventilated patients, keep positive end expiratory pressure as low as possible to decrease transpulmonary pressures and minimize right-ventricle afterload. Respiratory rate should be set low to avoid air trapping.

PHYSICAL EXAMINATION

- Tachycardia
- Hypotension
- Cyanosis
- Elevated jugular venous pressure (JVP) with large V waves
- RV heave
- Right-sided S_3
- Loud P2
- Parasternal heave
- Tricuspid regurgitation
- Pulsatile liver

DIFFERENTIAL DIAGNOSIS

- Myocardial infarction (MI)
- Complications of MI including intracardiac shunt, ruptured papillary muscle, ischemic MR
- Ventricular septal defect (VSD), atrial septal defect (ASD)
- Pulmonary embolus
- Pulmonary hypertension (primary or secondary)
- Congestive heart failure (CHF) exacerbation
- COPD exacerbation
- Pericardial disease

CAUSES OF RIGHT-VENTRICULAR FAILURE BY UNDERLYING PATHOPHYSIOLOGY

Pressure Overload
- Pulmonary embolus
- Left-sided heart failure
- Intracardiac shunt
- Pulmonic stenosis
- Pericardial disease
- Positive pressure ventilation
- Pulmonary hypertension
- Aortic or mitral valve disease
- Acute respiratory distress syndrome

Volume Overload
- Tricuspid regurgitation

- Pulmonic regurgitation
- Intracardiac shunt

Decreased Contractility
- RV infarction
- RV cardiomyopathy
- Peri-operative RV injury

Others
- Sepsis
- Congenital heart disease

DIAGNOSTIC TESTS

ECG, CXR, cardiac biomarkers show evidence of RV failure without infarction, including sinus tachycardia (ST), right-axis deviation, T-wave inversion in leads III, aVF or leads V1 to V4, deep S wave in lead I with T-wave inversion and Q wave in lead III, and Qr in lead V1. ECG signs of RV infarction include ST elevations and loss of R wave in V1 and in V3R and V4R. Chest radiography may show dilated pulmonary arteries, filling of the retrosternal space from RV enlargement, or increased curvature of the right-heart border. Troponin and BNP are important not only as diagnostic tools but also as prognostic indicators of outcome. Cardiac troponin levels are elevated in the setting of RV infarction but can also be elevated in RV dysfunction due to microinfarction or ischemia. BNP is synthesized as a result of RV shear stress and correlates with the degree of RV dysfunction. Thus, elevated cardiac biomarkers can identify high-risk patients.

Transthoracic echocardiography is an important diagnostic modality in the evaluation of a patient with suspected RV failure. Not only can RV dilatation and decreased function be seen, but valvular function, chamber size, hypertrophy, pulmonary artery dilation and pressure gradients, pericardial disease, and shunt can be assessed. In the parasternal short view, RV pressure overload can be seen as septal flattening during systole. RV volume overload is characterized by septal flattening during diastole with normalization of septal curvature during systole. *McConnell's sign* is an echocardiographic finding specific to pulmonary embolus with diffuse RV hypokinesis and sparing of the apex. Transesophageal echocardiographic (TEE) evaluation of the right ventricle may be necessary due to poor penetrance via a transthoracic approach in some individuals.

Pulmonary artery (PA) catheterization is useful in evaluating RV dysfunction in the intensive care unit (ICU) setting. Pulmonary pressures may be elevated due to pulmonary disease or left-sided heart failure. RV infarction is characterized by elevated RV pressures—specifically RV diastolic pressure signaling increased stiffness—and RA pressures but pulmonary artery pressures may not be elevated. Tricuspid regurgitation leads to elevated mean RA pressures with a broad C-V wave and exaggerated y descent. A depressed RV stroke volume can be estimated by a narrow pulmonary artery pulse pressure. The equalization of pressures can suggest pericardial constriction versus restriction. Last, a shunt run looking for an oxygen "step up" can diagnose a VSD or ASD if clinically suspected.

As discussed next, optimal preload conditions can be accurately assessed with PA catheterization and can guide fluid management. Pulmonary pressures and cardiac output can be measured and should be monitored if pressors, inotropes, or pulmonary vasodilators are used.

MEDICAL MANAGEMENT

The successful management of RV failure rests on treating the underlying disease process and supportive care. Examples are coronary revascularization for RV infarction, thrombolysis or embolectomy for pulmonary embolus, and tricuspid repair can be considered for severe tricuspid regurgitation. Supportive care includes the following:

Supplemental oxygen: Continuous oxygen therapy is essential in managing RV dysfunction especially in the setting of hypoxemia. While the etiology is being investigated, it is important to avoid hypoxia-induced vasoconstriction, worsening RV afterload. Intubation and mechanical ventilation may be required.

IV fluids: Patients with RV failure are often preload dependent, but fluid status is difficult to assess without PA catheterization. If CVP <12 mmHg, normal saline boluses may be administered for goal CVP 12 to 15 mmHg. If CVP >12 mmHg, additional fluids are not necessary.

Pressors and inotropes: Norepinephrine, vasopressin, or high-dose dopamine can be used to manage systemic hypotension. Inotropes improve contractility and hemodynamics. However, they may provoke or worsen systemic hypotension and may need to be used in conjunction with pressors. Dobutamine is the preferable inotrope of choice given its preferable side-effect profile compared to milrinone.

Diagnosis and Management of Pulmonary Embolus

Diagnosis:

- Massive PE is suspected in patients with evidence of right-ventricular failure, normal CXR, an ECG suggestive of right-ventricular strain, hypoxemia or elevated A-a gradient, and hypotension without other cause (e.g., arrhythmia, hypovolemia, sepsis).
- Cardiac biomarkers: Cardiac troponin and BNP are not helpful in diagnosis but are useful in risk stratification and prognosis
- CT with IV contrast or V/Q scan: should be obtained to confirm the diagnosis if the patient is stable.
- TEE can be used if the patient is too unstable for another imaging study and massive PE is suspected.
- TTE and lower extremity duplex ultrasound: Bedside procedures that can help with the diagnosis and management.

Management:

- Unfractionated heparin with bolus or low molecular weight heparin should be started immediately.

Thrombolysis

- Appropriate for patients who are hemodynamically compromised and can consider for hemodynamically "stable" patients with RV dilation and/or dysfunction
- Determine whether the patient has any contraindications
  - Absolute: history of hemorrhagic stroke, intracranial neoplasm, recent (<2 months) intracranial surgery or trauma, active or recent internal bleed in past 6 months
  - Relative: bleeding diathesis, uncontrolled hypertension (sbp >200 mmHg, dbp >110 mmHg), prolonged cardiopulmonary resuscitation, nonhemorrhagic stroke within past 2 months, surgery in past 10 days, thrombocytopenia (<10,000)
- If the patient has no contraindications, then thrombolysis should be administered
  - alteplase: 10 mg IV bolus, then 90 mg over 90 minutes
  - streptokinase: 250,000 U IV loading dose over 30 minutes, then 100,000 U/hr for 24 hours
  - reteplase: 10 U IV over 2 minutes, followed by 10 U IV 30 minutes later

Transvenous catheter embolectomy: Consider if the patient has contraindications to thrombolysis and is hemodynamically stable

Surgical embolectomy: Consider if the patient has contraindications to thrombolysis and is hemodynamically unstable

IVC filter: Should be placed if the patient has a deep venous thrombosis with contraindications to anticoagulation or if an embolic phenomenon from the lower extremities could be life threatening.

Selective pulmonary vasodilators: Prostacyclin and its analogs are not considered standard of care for RV dysfunction in general but have distinct roles in the treatment of pulmonary hypertension, which are discussed in Chapter 23. Inhaled nitric oxide (NO) has been investigated in a variety of conditions associated with acute RV dysfunction including RV infarction, acute respiratory distress syndrome (ARDS), and pulmonary embolus. Studies suggest improvement in pulmonary artery pressures, pulmonary vascular resistance, and increased cardiac output. Inhaled NO can be started at 10 ppm and can be titrated up by 10 ppm every 20 to 30 minutes to a maximum dose of 80 ppm.

IABP: Intra-aortic balloon counterpulsation can improve RV function by augmenting coronary blood flow and increasing systemic pressure, which can obviate the need for pressors. This approach is particularly relevant to the management of RV infarctions.

SURGICAL MANAGEMENT

Atrial septostomy: The creation of a shunt between the right and left atria leads to hypoxemia but decompresses the right side and augments filling of the left-sided chambers, leading to improved cardiac output and oxygen delivery. This is an option that is generally considered when all else has failed.

ECMO: Extracorporeal membrane oxygenation can be implemented if there is severe lung injury accompanying RV failure. This is considered if the underlying cause is reversible and if the patient has been ventilated for fewer than 5 days.

RVAD and consideration of transplant: In situations in which cardiac output remains low despite aggressive medical management, right ventricular assist devices (RVAD) can be considered for isolated RV failure as a bridge to transplant or less frequently, bridge-to-recovery or destination therapy. Biventricular failure is more common than isolated RV failure in which case biventricular assist device (BiVAD) support or total artifical heart (TAH) should be considered.

RECOMMENDED READING

1. Kucher N, Goldhaber SZ. Management of massive pulmonary embolism. *Circulation.* 2005; 112:e28–32.
2. McNeil K, Dunning J, NW Morrell. The pulmonary physician in critical care 13: the pulmonary circulation and right ventricular failure in the ITU. *Thorax.* 2003; 58:157–162.
3. Piazza G, Goldhaber SZ. The acutely decompensated right ventricle: pathways for diagnosis and management. *Chest.* 2005; 128:1836–1852.

CHAPTER 22

Pulmonary Hypertension

DEEPU S. NAIR

Pulmonary hypertension can be a feature of a variety of cardiopulmonary conditions, a complication of systemic disease, or a primary disorder of pulmonary vasculature. In the cardiac intensive care unit (CICU), elevated pulmonary artery pressure (PAP) most commonly results from pulmonary venous hypertension due to left-sided cardiac disease. Pulmonary arterial hypertension (PAH), defined as a resting mean pulmonary artery pressure >25 mmHg with normal pulmonary capillary wedge pressure (PCWP), can result from chronic hypoxemia, processes causing obstruction or destruction of the pulmonary vasculature, and a host of other disorders. PAH causes an increased pressure load on the right ventricle (RV) that initially triggers adaptive hypertrophy and dilatation. When the RV is no longer able to respond to the hemodynamic stress, RV failure and cor pulmonale can develop.

A growing body of research suggests that PAH results from vascular proliferation and remodeling at the level of the small pulmonary arteries. Specifically, increased pulmonary vascular resistance is thought to result from vasoconstriction, remodeling of the pulmonary vessel wall, and thrombosis in situ (Fig. 22.1). As the understanding of pulmonary hypertension has grown, a variety of new and promising therapies, including drugs such as bosentan and sildenafil, have become available for use in patients.

PRESENTATION

The onset of symptoms with PAH can be insidious, accounting for the long delay in diagnosis in most cases. Dyspnea, particularly with exertion, and generalized fatigue are the most common presenting symp-

ACUTE MANAGEMENT

Diagnostic Tests:

- **ECG:** right-atrial enlargement (P-pulmonale), right-axis deviation, right-ventricular hypertrophy with strain (tall R waves V1, V2 with repolarization abnormality), tachycardia, atrial arrhythmias
- **CXR:** right-ventricular enlargement, prominence of PAs, attenuation of peripheral pulmonary vascular markings, $+/-$ interstitial lung disease, $+/-$ emphysematous changes
- **TTE:** Evaluate left-ventricular function and valves. Assess right-ventricular contractility, size & hypertrophy, and estimate pulmonary artery systolic pressure (PASP) using triscupid regurgitation (TR) velocity (modified Bernoulli equation). Engorgement and noncompressibility of the inferior vena cava and presence of septal flattening suggest volume and/or pressure overload of the right ventricle.
- **Right Heart Catheterization:** In unstable patients or those in whom the contribution of left-sided heart disease to PAH remains uncertain, right heart cath can be useful as it provides measurements of PA pressure, pulmonary capillary wedge pressure, and cardiac output.
- **CT scan/MRI:** if suspicion for acute (or acute on chronic) pulmonary embolism exists, CT should be performed urgently. A V/Q scan may also be considered in this situation.

Management:

- **Tools:** Large-bore IV line and/or central line, arterial line, pulmonary artery catheter in acutely decompensated patient
- **STAT Labs:** CBC, CMP, PT, INR, PTT, type and screen, cardiac biomarkers

Medications:

- Oxygen: hypoxemia raises pulmonary vascular resistance (PVR); O_2 is a good pulmonary vasodilator
- $+/-$ gentle intravenous fluids (IVF): patients are preload dependent—ensure adequate volume
- Avoid venodilators and agents which reduce preload
- Administer nonselective vasodilators such as nitroprusside
- Nitric oxide can reduce PVR and improve hemodynamics
  - start at 10 ppm and titrate to 80 ppm

- Sildenafil can be considered for patients able to take medications by mouth
- Inotropes such as dobutamine can be considered to support right-ventricular function
- Heparin should be started if pulmonary embolism is suspected
  - Consider lytics for hemodynamically compromised patients without contraindications
  - alteplase 100 mg IV over 2 hours

CCU Tips: Maintaining preload is essential, but avoid overaggressive fluid resuscitation. Outcomes for patients with PAH are dismal if they arrest, even with rapid resuscitation. Transient elevations in PAP are often seen in patients with left-ventricular ischemia and dynamic changes in left-ventricular diastolic function. The right ventricle can only generate ~30–40 mmHg pressure acutely; higher pulmonary artery (PA) pressures indicate a more chronic process.

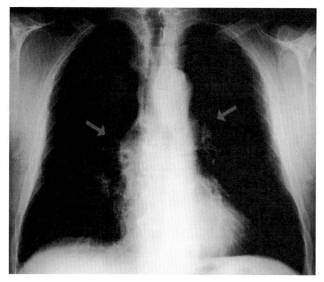

FIGURE 22.1. Chest x-ray of patient with PAH showing enlargement of central pulmonary arteries (arrows) and marked attenuation, or "pruning," of peripheral pulmonary vasculature.

toms for PAH. Angina and syncope can be present, and portend a worse prognosis. Signs of right-sided heart failure, such as peripheral edema or ascites, may be present. Rarely, hoarseness has been described due to compression of the recurrent laryngeal nerve by an enlarged pulmonary artery (Ortner's syndrome).

In patients with pulmonary hypertension associated with left-sided heart disease, there can be considerable overlap in symptoms attributed to left-heart failure and PAH, respectively. These patients may have concomitant signs of decreased cardiac output due to decreased left-ventricular (LV) function or left-sided valvular lesions.

PHYSICAL EXAMINATION

- General: tachypnea
- Neck: elevated jugular venous pressure (JVP), prominent V wave (due to TR), hepatojugular reflex
- Cardiac: resting tachycardia, TR murmur, RV heave, prominent P2 +/− palpable P2, +/− RV S3, rarely PI murmur, +/− signs of left-heart failure (if left-sided heart disease is etiology)
- Lungs: usually clear, +/− decreased breath sounds (if chronic obstructive pulmonary disease [COPD]), +/− fine crackles (if interstitial lung disease [ILD]), +/− crackles (if left-heart failure)
- Abdomen: hepatomegaly, pulsatile liver
- Extremities: peripheral edema, clubbing, +/− cyanosis

DIFFERENTIAL DIAGNOSIS

- Severe pulmonic stenosis or regurgitation
- Severe tricuspid stenosis or regurgitation
- RV myocardial infarction (MI)
- Acute pulmonary embolism
- Cardiac tamponade
- Restrictive cardiomyopathy
- Atrial septal defect (ASD), ventricular septal defect (VSD)
- Chronic obstructive pulmonary disease (COPD) exacerbation
- Pericardial disease

DIAGNOSTIC TESTS

The initial step in evaluating PAH is confirmation of the diagnosis, usually with transthoracic echocardiography. Interrogation of the TR jet

Causes of Pulmonary Hypertension

Cardiac	Left-heart abnormalities
	Cardiomyopathies
	Valvular heart disease
	Congenital heart disease
Pulmonary	Chronic obstructive pulmonary disease
	Interstitial lung disease
	Sleep-disordered breathing
	Alveolar hypoventilation disorders
	Chronic high-altitude exposure
Obstruction of	Chronic thromboembolic disease
Pulmonary vasculature	Nonthrombotic pulmonary embolism (e.g., tumor)
	Hemoglobinopathies
	Schistosomiasis
Collagen vascular	CREST
Disease	Scleroderma
Rheumatoid arthritis	
Toxins	Anorexic agents, crack cocaine
Familial	Genetic mutation (BMPR gene)
Idiopathic	Primary pulmonary hypertension
Miscellaneous	Infection—HIV
	Portal hypertension
	Pulmonary veno-occlusive disease

velocity allows estimation of PASP using the modified Bernouilli equation. Right-heart catheterization is done to confirm elevated pulmonary pressures and is useful for management of unstable patients. The range of other diagnostic tests available should be used to search for primary disorders that may be causing pulmonary hypertension. A careful evaluation of LV systolic and diastolic function as well as left-sided valvular function is critical, as left-sided heart disease is perhaps the most common cause of elevated PA pressure in the CICU. Serologic testing for evidence of underlying collagen vascular disease or autoimmune disease is also critically important.

ECG evidence of RV failure without infarction includes sinus tachycardia, right-axis deviation, T-wave inversion in leads III, aVF or leads

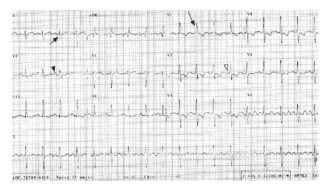

FIGURE 22.2. ECG of patient with advanced PAH. Features illustrated include right-axis deviation, P-pulmonale (lead II), and incomplete right branch bundle block with strain pattern (with permission from Naueser et al. *Am Fam Physician.* 2001; 63(9):10).

V1–V4, deep S wave in lead I with T-wave inversion and Q wave in lead III, and Qr in lead V1. ECG signs of RV infarction include ST elevations and loss of R wave in V1 and in V3R and V4R (Fig. 22.2).

CXR may show dilated pulmonary arteries, filling of the retrosternal space from RV enlargement, or increased curvature of the right-heart border.

Pulmonary artery catheterization is useful in evaluating RV dysfunction in the intensive care unit (ICU) setting. Pulmonary pressures may be elevated due to pulmonary disease or left-sided heart failure. RV infarction is characterized by elevated RV diastolic and right atrial pressures, but pulmonary artery pressures may not be elevated. Tricuspid regurgitation leads to elevated mean right-atrial pressures with a broad C–V wave and exaggerated y descent. A depressed RV stroke volume can be estimated by a narrow pulmonary artery pulse pressure. The equalization of pressures can suggest pericardial constriction versus restriction. Last, a shunt run looking for an oxygen "step up" can diagnose a VSD or ASD if clinically suspected.

Transthoracic echocardiography (TTE) should be performed soon after the patient's arrival to the ICU. Doppler measurements across the TV should be used to estimate PASP. Given the right ventricle's crescentic shape, several views are generally necessary to provide accurate estimates of right ventricle size, hypertrophy and systolic function. Septal flattening in diastole and/or systole suggests RV volume and pressure overload, as does inferior vena cava (IVC) plethora. Diffuse RV hypokinesis with apical sparing (McConnell's sign) may indicate a pulmonary embolism. LV systolic and diastolic function as well as left-sided valve function should be evaluated to identify any primary disorder that may account for pulmonary hypertension.

Computed tomography (CT) may suggest a cause of PAH, such as severe airway or parenchymal lung disease, and it can be performed once initial stabilization has occurred. The excellent spatial resolution of CT allows accurate measurement of right ventricle size, PA size and lung parenchyma. In the setting of chronic thromboembolic PAH, thrombus may be seen within the pulmonary arteries, though CT is relatively less sensitive than V/Q for chronic pulmonary embolism (PE).

Ventilation-perfusion (V/Q) remains a useful test in differentiating whether the cause of PAH is chronic thromboembolic disease, though its sensitivity is much higher than its specificity for this condition.

Magnetic imaging resonance (MRI) is emerging as a highly sensitive and specific test for chronic thromboembolism. In one study, sensitivity was 89% and specificity was 100% when measured against TTE as a gold standard. It also provides detailed information about RV function, valvular abnormalities, and lung parenchymal abnormalities.

Laboratory evaluation of patients with unexplained PAH should include ANA, TSH, liver function tests, and HIV testing in some cases.

MEDICAL MANAGEMENT

Initial attention should be focused on physical examination, including measurement of vital signs such as arm blood pressures, oxygen saturation, identification of jugular venous distention (JVD) and careful cardiac auscultation. Signs of right-sided heart failure such as edema, ascites, and elevated JVP may be present. Hypotension can indicate RV failure due to elevated PAP.

Two large-bore IV sites and a radial arterial line should be placed for administration of vasoactive medications and close hemodynamic monitoring, respectively. Consideration should be given to placement of a central venous catheter in unstable patients to allow rapid medication delivery.

A PA catheter can be useful for management of patients with hemodynamic compromise, as it may guide optimal titration of vasoactive medications.

Oxygen should be administered as it can produce pulmonary vasodilatation.

Anticoagulation in patients with idiopathic PAH is based on two small studies which reported improved survival, and its use in PAH due to congenital heart disease (CHD) or left-sided heart disease is less clear. Patients with suspected chronic or acute PE should be started on IV heparin while confirmatory studies are pursued.

Volume management in patients with RV failure can be complex with the goal being to optimize RV and LV preload. These patients may require a higher than normal preload, but on presentation may already be significantly volume overloaded. Thus a PA catheter can greatly guide therapy.

Pulmonary vasodilator therapy can be extremely useful. Vasodilator testing can be performed with a PA catheter. This is accomplished by taking baseline measurements, administering a vasodilator (nitric oxide, prostacyclin, adenosine), and monitoring change in PVR and PA pressure. If PA pressure is reduced by more than 10 mmHg to a value lower than 40 mmHg, the patient may have a good response to calcium-channel blocker (CCB) therapy. However, in unstable patients, short-acting agents such as prostacyclin or inhaled nitric oxide (NO) are preferred. In hypotensive patients, inhaled NO or iloprost are favored as their effects are limited to the pulmonary bed.

- **Intravenous prostacyclin (epoprostenol)** induces smooth muscle relaxation by stimulating cAMP production and has been shown in short-term trials to result in functional improvement. **Iloprost**, an inhaled prostacyclin analogue, and **treprostinil**, a subcutaneously infused prostacyclin, have also been shown to improve hemodynamic variables in PAH.
- **Bosentan** is effective in improving functional capacity, but its use can be limited by dose-dependent hepatic aminotransferase elevation (3%–7%).
- **Inhaled NO** is a potent vasodilator and is useful for short-term therapy.
- **Sildenafil**, a phosphodiesterase inhibitor, enhances NO-dependent vasodilation and can be utilized as an oral alternative.

In patients with **elevated PCWP and pulmonary hypertension**, treatment should be aimed at improving left-sided heart function and reducing PCWP. This can be accomplished with system vasodilator therapy with agents such as nitroprusside. Occasionally, ionotropes are necessary if hypotension is present. In refractory cases, an IABP may be used. In these patients with LV systolic or diastolic failure, specific PAH therapy should not be initiated until optimization of LV function with traditional chronic heart failure (CHF) therapies has occurred.

SURGICAL MANAGEMENT

In patients with thromboembolic PAH, pulmonary endarterectomy should be considered. The surgery can be potentially curative though the operative mortality remains near 5%. For patients who do not respond to conventional therapy and are appropriate candidates, lung or heart-lung transplant can be considered. Atrial septostomy, or creation of a right-to-left atrial shunt to offload RV pressure, can cause profound hypoxemia or pulmonary edema and is reserved as a palliative measure. Extracorporeal membrance oxygenation (ECMO) can be implemented if there is severe lung injury that is reversible accompanying the RV failure. Finally, an right-ventricle assist device (RVAD) may be considered if heart transplant is an option.

COMPLICATIONS

Right ventricular failure (cor pulmonale) is the eventual outcome of long-standing PAH and portends a poor prognosis. RV failure can result in severe hepatic congestion, ascites, and anasarca.

Syncope can be a manifestation of decreased cardiac output due to elevated PA pressure.

Hypotension must be combatted aggressively to prevent systemic pressures from dropping below pulmonary pressures.

DISCHARGE

The patient with pulmonary hypertension can be safely discharged from the ICU once hemodynamic stability has been achieved, and an adequate medical regimen for management of PA pressures has been instituted. In some cases, pulmonary vasodilator testing as previously described will allow treatment with CCB's; alternatively, therapy with agents such as bosentan or sildenafil may have been instituted. In either case, adequate response to these drugs in terms of both PA pressure and symptoms should be documented prior to ICU discharge. Long-term therapy with oxygen and anticoagulation should be instituted in most patients. For patients with left-sided heart disease, transition from IV vasodilators to oral agents such as ACE-I should be accomplished while in the ICU.

RECOMMENDED READING

1. Runo JR, Loyd JE. *Primary Pulmonary Hypertension.* Lancet; 2003; 361 (9368):1533–1544.
2. Rubin LJ, Primary pulmonary hypertension. *N Engl J Med.* 1997; 336(2): 111–117.
3. Humbert M, Sitbon O, Simonneau G. Treatment of pulmonary arterial hypertension. *N Engl J Med.* 2004; 351(14):1425–1436.
4. Rubin LJ, Badesch DB. Evaluation and management of the patient with pulmonary arterial hypertension. *Ann Intern Med.* 2005; 143(4):282–292.
5. Kruger S, et al. Diagnosis of pulmonary arterial hypertension and pulmonary embolism with magnetic resonance angiography. *Chest.* 2001; 120(5): 1556–1561.
6. Rich S, Kaufmann E, Levy PS. The effect of high doses of calcium-channel blockers on survival in primary pulmonary hypertension. *N Engl J Med.* 1992; 327(2):76–81.
7. Fuster V, et al. Primary pulmonary hypertension: natural history and the importance of thrombosis. *Circulation.* 1984; 70(4):580–587.
8. Barst RJ, et al. A comparison of continuous intravenous epoprostenol (prostacyclin) with conventional therapy for primary pulmonary hypertension. The Primary Pulmonary Hypertension Study Group. *N Engl J Med,* 1996; 334(5):296–302.
9. Raiesdana A, Loscalzo J. Pulmonary arterial hypertension. *Ann Med,* 2006; 38(2):95–110.
10. Nauser TD, Stites SW. *Diagnosis and treatment of pulmonary hypertension. Am Fam Physician.* 2001; 63(9):1789–1798.

CHAPTER **23**

Hypertrophic Cardiomyopathy

MEHDI H. SHISHEHBOR

Hypertrophic cardiomyopathy (HCM) results from significant myocardial hypertrophy with and without significant obstruction in the absence of an identifiable cause.

PRESENTATION

Patients may present with (a) syncope and presyncope caused by inadequate cardiac output and poor cerebral perfusion; (b) myocardial ischemia usually as a result of supply and demand mismatch; (c) heart failure secondary to dynamic outflow tract obstruction and diastolic dysfunction; (d) sudden death. Any process that increases heart rate, decreases preload, shortens diastolic filling time, worsens left-ventricular (LV) compliance (i.e., ischemia), and increases LV outflow obstruction (i.e., tachyarrhythmias and exercise) can lead to cardiac intensive care unit (CICU) admission for these patients.

PHYSICAL EXAMINATION

- Laterally displaced apical impulse
- Palpable S_4
- Bifid pulse and rapid carotid upstroke
- Harsh, cresendo-decresendo holosystolic murmur at the left sternal boarder
- Any condition or medication that decreases preload (venous return) or decreases systemic vascular resistance increases hypertrophic cardiomyopathy (HCM) murmur (i.e., Valsalva, standing, amyl nitrite, extrasystole)

212

ACUTE MANAGEMENT

Diagnostic Tests:

- **ECG:** To assess for evidence of ischemia
- **TTE:** To diagnose hypertrophic cardiomyopathy, determine the cause, location, severity, and examine the presence of systolic anterior motion of the mital valve
- Look for enlarged septum
- Continuous wave doppler flow of left-ventricular outflow tract with resting gradient of >30 mmHg or >50 mmHg with provocation (i.e., valsalva) confirms the diagnosis

Management:

- **Tools:** Two large-bore IV lines
- **STAT labs:** Type and cross, CBC, CMP, ECG, portable CXR, PT, INR, PTT, and cardiac enzymes

Medications:

- In the setting of a tachyarrhythmia, utilize:
  - IV Metoprolol 5 mg q5 to 10 minutes until heart rate 50–60, if not in acute heart failure
  - IV Diltiazem 0.25 mg/kg over 2 minutes, if no response in 5–10 minutes then repeat loading with 0.35 mg/kg, maintenance dose 5–15 mg/hour, use if there is contraindication to beta-blocker therapy, avoid in acute heart failure
  - Disopyramide 300–400 mg initial oral dose than 2–4 mg/min, if beta-blocker and calcium-channel blocker therapy are unsuccessful
  - DC cardioversion if the patient is unstable (with atrial fibrillation/flutter)
- For pulmonary edema and hypotension
  - Judicious IV lasix for pulmonary congestion
  - phenylepherine 0.5–15 µg/kg/min in rare situations—please see below

Surgical: Surgical or percutaneous consideration

CCU Tip: If patient develops chest pain, consider beta blockers. Extreme caution with nitrate use.

DIFFERENTIAL DIAGNOSIS

- Yamaguchi's apical HCM patients present with chest pain, dyspnea, and fatigue. Most commonly seen in Japan.
- HCM of the elderly—Associated with hypertension
- Secondary HCM (i.e., prolong hypertension)
- Aortic stenosis
- Supravalvular aortic stenosis (AS): Associated with William's syndrome
- Subvalvular AS: Fibromuscular membrane located in the left-ventricular outflow tract (LVOT)

RISK FACTORS

- Familial transmission
- Myosin heavy chain mutation (14q1)—most common
- Cardiac troponin T mutation (1q31)
- Family history of sudden cardiac death

DIAGNOSTIC TESTS

Transthoracic echocardiography is used to diagnose HCM using the following criteria: (Adopted from Griffin and Topol)

- Asymmetric septal hypertrophy (>13 mm) (Fig. 23.1)
- Ratio of septal to posterior wall thickness of 1.3 or greater (nonhypertensive patients), 1.5 or greater (hypertensive patients)
- Systolic anterior motion of the mitral valve (SAM)—caused by Venturi effect of high-flow velocity through the narrow outflow tract (Fig. 23.2)
- Small LV cavity
- Septal immobility
- Premature closure of the aortic valve
- Resting gradient >30 mmHg
- Provacable gradients >50 mmHg
- Reduced rate of closure of the mitral valve in mid-diastole
- Mitral valve prolapse with regurgitation
- Maximal LV diastolic wall thickness >15 mm
- Dagger appearance of mitral valve on M-mode echocardiography (Fig. 23.3)

Magnetic resonance imaging (MRI) produces three-dimensional imaging with excellent resolution and tissue characterization.

Cardiac catheterization, required for almost all patients undergoing myectomy, shows the following characteristic findings: (Adopted from Griffin and Topol)

- Subaortic or midventricular outflow gradient on catheter pullback
- Spike-and-dome pattern of aortic pressure tracing as a consequence of outlet obstruction
- Elevated right- and left-ventricular (LV) end-diastolic pressures
- Elevated pulmonary capillary wedge pressure (PCWP)
- Increased V wave on wedge tracing (Fig. 23.3) Elevated pulmonary arterial pressure
- Brockenbrough's sign (Fig. 23.4) (the pulse pressure fails to widen in a beat following a premature ventricular beat)

MEDICAL MANAGEMENT

Initial physical exam of the patient should include a full cardiac and pulmonary exam to assess volume status and precipitating factors.

A minimum of two large-bore IV sites and a type and screen sent with preliminary laboratory studies.

The goal in patients with HCM is to maintain adequate volume status while minimizing diastolic and systolic dysfunction. Special attention should be given to conditions that increase myocardial contractility

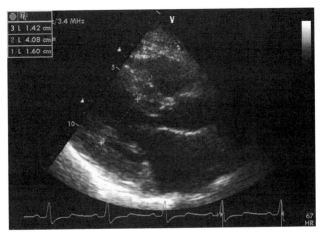

FIGURE 23.1. Parasternal long-axis view of a hypertrophic heart.

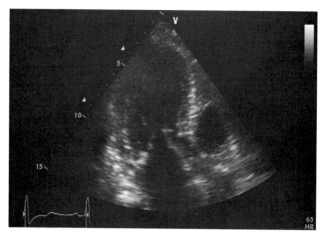

FIGURE 23.2. Apical view of systolic anterior motion of the mitral valve causing LVOT obstruction.

and diminish diastolic filling time (i.e., atrial fibrillation, tachyarrhythmias, ischemia, thyroid dysfunction, sepsis, and volume shift). Beta blockers are first-line therapy as they decrease myocardial oxygen demand and increase diastolic filling time. IV metoprolol 5 mg every 5 minutes for a goal heart rate of 50 to 60 should be sufficient. If beta blocker use is contraindicated, IV diltiazem can be used. Occasionally,

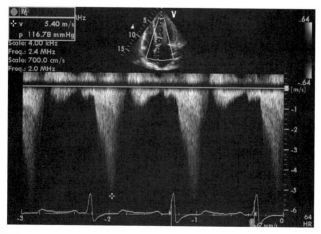

FIGURE 23.3. Characteristic dagger-shaped continuous-wave Doppler flow through the LVOT.

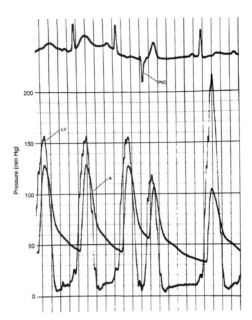

FIGURE 23.4. Brockenbrough's sign.

patients may require disopyramide, a class 1A antiarrhythmic agent. It is a potent negative inotropic agent; however, it is associated with significant anticholinergic properties that make its use undesirable. Avoid in patients with atrial fibrillation as it may enhance atrioventricular nodal conduction. Dose should be adjusted in the presence of renal or hepatic dysfunction. On rare occasions use phenylephrine to decrease LV outflow tract gradient in patients with no evidence of myocardial ischemia who are still symptomatic despite adequate volume resuscitation, beta blocker, calcium channel blockers, and disopyramide use. If the patient is hemodynamically unstable with a rapid atrial fibrillation, DC cardioversion should be considered.

Alcohol ablation, currently indicated for patients deemed poor surgical candidates, is occasionally associated with heart block; therefore, these patients typically have temporary pacemakers and are monitored in the ICU for 24 to 48 hours.

SURGICAL MANAGEMENT

Patients with symptomatic HCM require immediate surgical or alcohol septal ablation.

CLINICAL PRESENTATION TIPS

- Hypotension: Suspect volume depletion, increased outflow gradient, or ischemia.
- Acute MI: CAD, myocardial bridging, mismatch of supply and demand.
- Respiratory Distress: Acute heart failure.
- Arrhythmias/Heart block: Any arrhythmia that may increase oxygen demand or decrease diastolic filling time/volume (i.e., atrial fibrillation).
- Mental status change: Associated with exertion and decreased cardiac output.
- Decreased Urine Output: Associated with decreased cardiac output.
- Syncope/presyncope: Occasionally associated with exertion and decreased cardiac output.
- Sudden Death: Associated risk factors include family history of sudden death, sustained ventricular tachycardia, prior cardiac arrest, multiple nonsustained ventricular tachycardia on monitoring, abnormal decrease in exercise blood pressure, resting left-ventricular outflow tract obstruction >30 mmHg, and recurrent syncope or exertional near syncope (adopted from Griffin and Topol).

COMPLICATIONS

Syncope and presyncope—patients with HCM are preload dependent. Initial step in evaluating patients with HCM is to assess volume status. In addition, these patients are at an increased risk of sudden cardiac death; therefore a careful history and physical exam should be performed to assess the cause of syncope. An ICD may be considered in individuals with genetic predisposition for sudden cardiac death.

Myocardial ischemia can be secondary to obstructive or nonobstructive coronary artery disease (CAD). It is most commonly associated with a mismatch of supply and demand. It may be related to increased myocardial wall tension, decreased capillary to myocardial fiber ratio, decreased coronary perfusion pressures, or myocardial bridging. Avoid drugs that decrease preload (i.e., nitrates) or decrease afterload (hydralazine).

Arrhythmias/heart block can have a profound impact on symptoms. Patients with HCM have very low reserve and are preload dependent. Any arrhythmia such as atrial fibrillation that impacts preload or increases oxygen demand will have a deleterious effects. Therefore, all arrhythmias should be treated very aggressively. If hemodynamic compromise or end-organ damage is present, cardioversion is the treatment of choice followed by appropriate IV drugs to prevent recurrence (e.g., IV sotalol or disopyramide). Avoid long-term Amiodarone use as it is associated with multiple side effects.

End-organ involvement may be associated with a low-output state leading to syncope and renal insufficiency. In the acute setting attention should be given to preload, diastolic filling time, and decreasing outflow gradient.

DISCHARGE

Patients with HCM can be transferred out of the intensive care unit (ICU) once they are hemodynamically stable. In addition, underlying reasons for their admission (i.e., atrial fibrillation, spesis, and dehydration) should have been addressed and resolved. In severe cases patients may need to be kept in the CICU until the obstruction is relieved either surgically or percutaneously.

RECOMMENDED READING

1. Wigle ED, Rakowski H, Kimball BP, et al. Hypertrophic cardiomyopathy. Clinical spectrum and treatment. *Circulation*. 1995; 92:1680–1692.
2. Maron BJ. Hypertrophic cardiomyopathy: a systematic review. *JAMA*. 2002; 287:1308–1320.
3. Nishimura RA, Holmes DR, Jr. Clinical practice. Hypertrophic obstructive cardiomyopathy. *N Engl J Med*. 2004; 350:1320–1327.

Mechanical Circulatory Support and Cardiac Transplantation

MICHAEL G. DICKINSON

Mechanical circulatory support (MCS) is beneficial in severely decompensated heart failure patients as a bridge to cardiac transplantation, as destination therapy (destination left-ventricular assist device [LVAD]), and in some cases as a bridge to recovery (especially from an acute insult). Cardiac transplantation results in a marked improvement in survival and quality of life and should be considered in patients with advanced chronic (AHA/ACC stage D, NYHA class III and IV) heart failure.

DIAGNOSTIC TESTS

Laboratory tests in patients being considered for mechanical circulatory support or cardiac transplantation start with basic studies evaluating for end organ dysfunction. These include a comprehensive metabolic panel (CMP), complete blood count (CBC), thyroid panel (TSH, free T3, free T4), urinalysis (UA) and coagulation studies (PT, PTT) and a B-type natriuretic peptide (BNP). Patients having a formal transplant evaluation will have a variety of metabolic, infectious disease, and allogen labs drawn (see table below).

Swan-Ganz catheter is essential for verifying and potentially diagnosing the etiology of shock. Patients with an elevated pulmonary capillary wedge pressure (PCWP) and inadequate CI (<2) with hypotension may be considered for MCS or transplant.

Coronary angiography evaluates for ischemia or viability, thus determining the etiology of cardiogenic shock and whether there are potential alternative therapies.

ACUTE MANAGEMENT

Indications for mechanical circulatory support (MCS):

- Massive myocardial infarction
- Acute myocarditis (especially giant cell myocarditis)
- Inability to wean patients from cardiopulmonary bypass (postcardiotomy cardiogenic shock)
- Previous cardiac transplantation with cardiogenic shock presumably due to graft failure (possible vascular rejection).

Other suggestions that a patient awaiting transplant will require MCS:

- Persistent low output state or evidence of impaired organ perfusion despite high dose or dual inotropic therapy.
- Hypotension or tachycardia in a patient on inotropic support.
- Elevation of pulmonary pressures despite maximal therapy with vasodilators and inotropes and efforts to optimize fluid status.
- Anticipated long-wait duration for transplant in a patient with marginal hemodynamics or organ perfusion.

Management:

- Telemetry, IV, access, supplemental oxygen, PA catheter
- Consider IABP if patient in cardiogenic shock or deteriorating
- **Stat Labs:** CBC, CMP, PT, INR, PTT, ECG, CXR, HSV 1&2, HVZ and transplant laboratory work-up including LFTs, TFTs, Type and Screen, CMV, toxoplasmosis, hepatitis B and C, HIV, and HLA tissue typing analysis
- **Studies:** Coronary angiography, carotid ultrasound, and abdominal ultrasound
- **Consults:** Obtain a transplant consult as a psychosocial assessment will be necessary to confirm the patient's suitability for mechanical circulatory support and potentially transplantation
- Rule out psychosocial inhibitors such as ongoing substance abuse, medical noncompliance, lack of psychosocial support, or prohibitive psychiatric problems
- LVAD therapies (implement with transplant specialist input):
  - Criteria for candidates for LVAD as bridge to transplant:
  - Patient is a transplant candidate

- Evidence of cardiogenic shock (Pulmonary capillary wedge pressure >20 mmHg, CI <2 L/min/m^2, and/or SBP ≤90 mmHg)
    - No exclusions (see below)
- Criteria for candidates for destination LVAD (DT-VAD)
    - Patient is not a transplant candidate
    - Patient is felt to have the adequate social support
    - Similar hemodynamic criteria as above (PCWP >20, CI <2, SBP ≤90).

CCU Tip: Patients should be considered early for mechanical support and the transplant team should be contacted as early as possible. If the patient has a high likelihood of successfully being bridged to recovery (e.g., stunned myocardium), mechanical circulatory support might be considered in a patient who is not otherwise a transplant or DT-VAD candidate.

VAD / TAH Exclusions:

1. Technical factors = BSA <1.5 m^2 (for implanted devices), significant Aortic insufficiency, R to L shunts, AAA, Prosthetic valves, LV thrombus
2. Severe right-ventricular failure: would require use of a BiVAD or TAH
3. Psychosocial factors that would result in poor patient compliance or inability to manage the device
4. Severe central nervous system depression (e.g., hypoxic encephalopathy)

Mechanical circulatory support telative contraindications: Patients who are at higher risk for perioperative complications including:

1. RAP >16 (i.e., impaired right-ventricular function): In these patients, consideration should be given for TAH or BiVAD (especially if there is a low right-ventricular stroke work index).
2. Coagulopathy (Prothrombin time >16)
3. Reoperation
4. Elevated white blood cell count (>15) or temperature >101.5°F
5. Urine output <30 cc/hr
6. Patients requiring positive pressure ventilation.

Carotid ultrasound/abdominal ultrasound evaluates for peripheral vascular disease, which must be worked up and excluded or treated prior to transplant.

Transplant consultation evaluates patients from a psychosocial perspective to determine whether they have factors that would prohibit MCS or transplant such as active substance abuse, medical noncompliance, or psychiatric disorders.

MECHANICAL CIRCULATORY SUPPORT (MCS)

A variety of technologies are used for MCS including intra-aortic balloon pumps (IABP), extracorporeal membrane oxygenation (ECMO), ventricular assist devices (VADs), total artificial hearts (TAHs) and a number of evolving technologies.

Intra-aortic Balloon Pump (IABP)

The IABP balloon is percutaneously placed via femoral arterial access into the descending thoracic aorta. The balloon is timed to inflate in diastole, with optimal balloon inflation starting at the arterial pressure waveform dicrotic notch (indicating aortic valve closure) and ending before the initiation of systole. IABPs provide effective afterload reduction and improved organ perfusion by augmenting diastolic flow. IABPs are indicated in heart failure with low output states unresponsive to inotropes and are contraindicated in aortic insufficiency, aortic dissection, and severe aortoiliac atherosclerosis. Please refer to Chapter 29 for further details.

Extracorporeal Membrane Oxygenation (ECMO)

ECMO involves surgical placement of large central venous and arterial cannulae. The ECMO system consists of a blood pump, a membrane oxygenator (which also removes carbon dioxide), and a countercurrent heat exchanger. ECMO is utilized for short-term (3–5 days) support of patients with severely impaired oxygenation or circulation when the patient is too ill to undergo VAD/TAH surgery. ECMO can be utilized in cardiac-arrest situations for acute percutaneous support at the bedside or in the cardiac catheterization laboratory. ECMO requires full anticoagulation and thus any coagulopathy must be considered prior to incorporation.

Ventricular Assist Devices (VADs)

VADs are primarily used for left-ventricular support (LVAD), but can be used for right-ventricular support (RVAD) or two devices can be used for biventricular support (BiVAD). For RVADs, the blood is drawn from the right atrium and channeled to the main pulmonary artery. For LVADs the blood is drawn from either the left atrium or the left-ventricle (LV) apex and channeled into the ascending aorta. Devices can be intracorporeal (inside the body) or extracorporeal (blood inflow and outflow lines exit the body to an external pump). Because of size limitations, a BiVAD generally requires at least one extracorporeal device. There are two basic classes of VADs: pulsatile flow (pneumatic and electric) and continuous flow (centrifugal or axial flow). Most devices require systemic anticoagulation (antiplatelet and antithrombotic) with device-specific anticoagulation protocols.

Pulsatile Flow Extracorporeal Devices

Abiomed BVS 5000   The BVS 5000 is FDA approved for short-term use (up to 7 days) for postcardiotomy shock. This is often used as a rescue device when patients are unable to be weaned from cardiopulmonary bypass at open heart surgery. The BVS 5000 can be changed to the Abiomed AB5000 ventricle (VAD) using the same cannulae if longer term support becomes necessary.

Thoratec VAD   The Thoratec VAD is a durable device and therefore is FDA approved for long-term use. It is often used in small patients (e.g., body surface area <1.5 m?) who cannot tolerate an intracorporeal device (or as an RVAD in patients needing BiVADs).

Pulsatile Flow Intracorporeal Devices

Novacor LVAS   The Novacor LVAS is electrically driven, with good implant experience demonstrating durability and is therefore a preferred device when long-term support is desired (such as in destination therapy). Anticoagulation is required and recent modifications of the cannulae have reduced the risk of thromboembolic complications.

Heartmate   The Heartmate IP is pneumatically driven and the Heartmate XVE (externally vented electric) is powered by an internal electric motor with transcutaneous drive lines consisting of electrical supply lines and a pneumatic venting tube (Fig. 24.1). It features a sintered titanium housing to promote rapid adherence of blood elements and formation of a pseuodointimal lining, which minimizes thromboembolism and therefore does not require long-term anticoagulation.

Continuous Flow Devices

All currently available continuous flow devices are investigational and not available outside of clinical trials. The devices can utilize axial flow

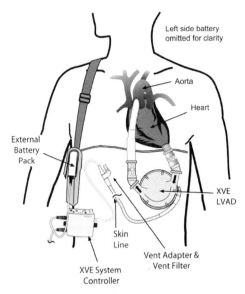

Left side battery omitted for clarity

Aorta

Heart

External Battery Pack

XVE LVAD

Skin Line

Vent Adapter & Vent Filter

XVE System Controller

FIGURE 24.1. Heartmate XVE LVAS. (Reprinted courtesy of the Thoratec Corporation.)

(Heartmate II, Jarvik2000 LVAD, MicroMed, Debakey VAD), in which a turbine like action is used to propel blood, or centrifugal flow (Kriton, and Ventracor Ventrassist) in which blood enters the center of the pump and is propelled to the outflow on the periphery of the pump. Although flow is continuous, output is preload dependent, so flow increases during right-ventricular (RV) systole because of increased supply to the pump. This often results in persistence of central arterial pulsatile flow. These devices have the advantage of smaller size, making them feasible in patients with smaller-body surface area. The Ventracor Ventrassist has been designed with a hydrodynamically suspended impeller and therefore has no bearings to theoretically be associated with greater reliability and wear.

Short-Term Percutaneously Placed Support Devices

CardiacAssist TandemHeart
The TandemHeart is an extracorporeal centrifugal continuous-flow pump that is placed percutaneously. Blood is removed from the left atrium and pumped to the distal aorta. The left-atrial supply line is placed via transseptal puncture to the left atrium using standard femoral venous access. The extracorporeal pump is fastened to the thigh, and a

return line is passed via the femoral artery to the distal aorta. It is indicated for short-term hemodynamic stabilization of patients in acute heart failure and for circulatory support during high-risk cardiac interventions. It can deliver outputs of up to 4 L/min. It can provide an alternative to ECMO in patients too ill to undergo VAD surgery but who have adequate oxygenation.

Impella Recover LD/LP 5.0 Support System
The Impella Recover is a high-speed (33,000 rpm) impeller pump located within a 9 Fr catheter. The catheter can be surgically placed directly in the left ventricle or percutaneously via the fermoral vein. It is currently in clinical development for short-term (up to 7 days) hemodynamic support as a bridge to more definitive therapy (such as VAD).

Total Artificial Hearts
Total artificial hearts are designed to replace both RV and LV function. They provide an intracorporeal solution for patients requiring biventricular support (all current BiVAD configurations require at least one extracorporeal device). The Syncardia Cardiowest TAH is approved for bridge to transplantation. The Abiocor TAH is currently investigational.

COMPLICATIONS

- **Peri-operative complications**—VAD/TAH patients face the same risks as patients undergoing any major cardiothoracic surgery.
- **Infection**—The rate of infection in patients with LVAD implantation as a bridge to transplantation can be as high as 50%. LVAD associated infection, however, is not a contraindication to transplant as patients may clear the infection once the device is removed.
- **Ventricular arrhythmias**—the device can irritate the left ventricle and precipitate arrhythmias in 25% of the patients
- **Left-ventricular thrombus**—the LVAD causes a thrombogenic environment; this occurs more commonly in postmyocardial infarction patients
- **HLA antigen sensitization**—Patients on MCS often require transfusion and, therefore, may develop elevated plasma reactive antigen (PRA) panels making it more difficult to locate an appropriate donor heart for transplantation.
- **Hemolytic anemia**—Hemolysis may occur due to red blood cell damage from the mechanical circuitry.
- **Thrombocytopenia**

DISCHARGE

Patients warranting MCS should only be discharged from the ICU after they are stabilized and do not have significant hemodynamic shifts. They require close evaluation for infection and anticoagulation. These patients may often be observed in the hospital while awaiting their transplant.

Cardiac Transplantation

Cardiac transplantation is performed in about 4,000 patients each year worldwide. The average survival posttransplantation is about 88% at 1 year, 70% at 5 years, and 50% at 10 years, making it an excellent option in patients with severe refractory heart failure. Given the limited donor supply, good outcomes are obtained with careful patient selection, meticulous follow up, and performing the procedure at a high-volume transplant center.

Cardiac Transplant Evaluation

Indications:

Severe refractory heart failure despite optimal medical management
Anticipated poor 1-year survival (based on clinical factors, MVO2 <14 or
    MVO2 <12 in a patient on beta blockers)
Recurrent malignant arrhythmias refractory to antiarrhythmic drugs or ablative
    techniques
Severe refractory angina refractory to all other therapies

Contraindications:

Advanced age (e.g., anticipated <10-year survival, age >65 is a relative con-
    traindication)
Irreversible end organ dysfunction (e.g., renal failure, cirrhosis)
Fixed pulmonary hypertension (>4 Woods units despite aggressive vasodilata-
    tion, inotropic or mechanical circulatory support)
Severe obstructive or restrictive pulmonary disease (not thought to be related to
    the heart failure or reversible by cardiac transplantation)
Significant peripheral vascular or cerebrovascular disease
Diabetic complications (retinopathy, nephropathy, neuropathy)
Ongoing tobacco and/or alcohol use
History of substance use (unless participation in rehabilitation and documented
    sustained abstinence)

Morbid Obesity

Psychiatric or psychosocial factors likely to result in noncompliance or which might decompensate on therapy with steroids.

Malignancy (active or recent without proof of cure [generally should be cancer free >5 years])

Any condition that would result in ongoing poor quality of life (e.g., severe neurologic disease or other disabilities).

Cardiac Transplant Exclusions:

— Advanced age (e.g., anticipated <10 year survival, age >65 is a relative contraindication)
— Irreversible end organ dysfunction (e.g., renal failure, cirrhosis)
— Fixed pulmonary hypertension (>4 Woods units despite aggressive vasodilatation, inotropic or mechanical circulatory support)
— Severe obstructive or restrictive pulmonary disease (not thought to be related to the heart failure or reversible by cardiac transplantation)
— Significant peripheral vascular or cerebrovascular disease
— Diabetic complications (retinopathy, nephropathy, neuropathy)
— Ongoing tobacco and/or alcohol use
— History of substance use (unless participation in rehabilitation and documented sustained abstinence)
— Obesity (e.g., body mass index >32)
— Psychiatric or psychosocial factors likely to result in noncompliance or which might decompensate on therapy with steroids.
— Malignancy (active or recent without proof of cure [generally should be cancer free >5 years])
— Any condition that would result in ongoing poor quality of life (e.g., severe neurologic disease or other disabilities).

Adult Transplantation Candidate Status

Status 1A	Inpatient + mechanical support, or intensive care unit patient with PA catheter on high dose or dual inotropes (life expectancy <7 days).
Status 1B	Ventricular assist device >30 days or continuous inotrope therapy not meeting above criteria.
Status 2	Does not meet status 1A or 1B criteria.
Status 7	Unsuitable to receive organ.

RECOMMENDED READING

1. Merhi W, Dixon SR, O'Neill WW, et al. Percutaneous left ventricular assist device in acute myocardial infarction and cardiogenic shock. *Rev Cardiovasc Med.* 2005; 6:118–123.

2. Simon D, Fischer S, Grossman A, et al. Left ventricular assist device-related infection: treatment and outcome. *Clin Infect Dis.* 2005; 40:1108–1115.
3. Herrmann M, Weyand M, Greshake B, et al. Left ventricular assist device infection is associated with increased mortality but is not a contraindication to transplantation. *Circulation.* 1997; 95:814–817.
4. Mancini D, Burkhoff D. Mechanical device-based methods of managing and treating heart failure. *Circulation.* 2005; 112:438–448.
5. Cimato TR, Jessup M. Recipient selection in cardiac transplantation: contraindications and risk factors for mortality. *J Heart Lung Transplant.* 2002; 21:1161–1173.

Management of the Acutely Decompensated Cardiac Transplant Patient

MICHAEL G. DICKINSON

In spite of increasingly sophisticated immunosuppression regimens, between 30% to 40% of transplant patients will experience an episode of moderate or severe rejection requiring treatment. Prompt recognition and treatment of rejection is of paramount importance in managing these patients.

PRESENTATION

The presentation of acute cardiac rejection can be highly variable. Patients may be asymptomatic or may be in frank cardiogenic shock with pulmonary edema. A high level of clinical suspicion must be held for patients with heart transplants presenting with signs or symptoms.

PHYSICAL EXAMINATION

- Fever
- Constitutional symptoms
- Hypotension may indicate graft failure
- Baseline neurologic exam to rule out central nervous system infections
- Evaluate for cardiac arrhythmia

DIFFERENTIAL DIAGNOSIS

Possible Triggers for Acute Cardiac Allograft Rejection
- Medication noncompliance

A C U T E   M A N A G E M E N T

Diagnostic Tests:

- Endomyocardial biopsy as early as possible
- Echocardiogram to evaluate for depressed ventricular function
- Right heart catheterization to monitor hemodynamics and cardiac output
- 12-lead ECG and telemetry to monitor for signs of cardiac irritability

Management:

- Telemetry, IV access, and supplemental oxygen as needed
- **Stat Labs:** CBC, CMP, PT, INR, PTT, CXR, ECG, blood culture, UA C&S, monitor immunosuppression levels (i.e., cyclosporine level, mycophenolate level) and check for CMV antigenemia; have a low threshold to evaluate for atypical infections
- Send biopsy samples for immunofluorescence or immunoperoxidase staining to rule out antibody mediated rejection and cellular rejection
- Therapies (implement in conjunction with transplant specialist input):
  - Discontinue any p450 interacting medications
  - Optimize anti-rejection medications based on levels
  - Consider pulse steroids (methylprednisolone 1,000 mg daily)
  - Consider cytolytic therapy with antithymocyte globulin or OKT3
  - Plasmapheresis if antibody mediated rejection
  - Consider heparin for microvascular thrombosis
  - Consider broad spectrum antibiotics if suspicious for infection
  - May need to use Dopamine or other ionotrope /pressors

CCU Tip: Have a very low threshold for invasive hemodynamic monitoring or aggressive infectious disease treatment and work-up for symptoms.

- Concomitant medications with P450 interactions resulting in subtherapeutic immunosuppressant medication levels
- Acute illness (especially cytomegalovirus [CMV] infection, but other viral or bacterial illnesses as well)
- Too rapid of steroid taper

Types of Rejection

Hyperacute Rejection

Hyperacute rejection is a violent, usually lethal immune response to the graft. It occurs immediately after transplantation (within minutes to hours) and is triggered by preformed antibodies to the graft. It generally presents as marked hemodynamic compromise that progresses to death. Fortunately, with the currently utilized cross-matching techniques, hyperacute rejection occurs quite rarely.

Acute Rejection

Acute cell mediated rejection is characterized by a mononuclear cell inflammatory response consisting mostly of lymphocytes. Donor and recipient antigen presenting cells interact with T-lymphocytes. The T-cells then release a variety of cytokines, which stimulate clonal T-cell proliferation, macrophage recruitment and activation, increased endothelial vascular permeability, and further cytokine activation. The end result is myocyte injury and necrosis. The severity of cell mediated rejection is graded by histological findings on endomyocardial biopsy (Table 25.1).

Antibody mediated rejection (AMR, previously known as humoral or vascular rejection) happens when antibodies directed at the donor vascular endothelial cells result in immunoglobulin/complement mediated injury to the cardiac microvasculature. The arteritis and venulitis results in endothelial cell activation, increased vascular permeability (with substantial myocardial tissue edema), alterations in antithrombin III, tissue plasminogen activator (TPA), and plasminogen activator inhibitor-1 (PAI-1) (with resultant microvascular thrombosis). Graft dysfunction with signs and symptoms of hemodynamic compromise are common. AMR is best diagnosed by immunoflourescence or immunoperoxidase staining for immunoglobulin (IgG, IgM or IgA), and complement (C3d, C4d, C1q), which are detected along the endothelial surfaces.

Chronic Rejection

Chronic rejection is a term applied to coronary allograft vasculopathy (CAV). CAV is one of the leading causes of late graft loss and results from diffuse intimal thickening of the coronary vasculature. This results in diffuse and widespread coronary artery disease and ischemic graft dysfunction that does not respond to usual revascularization techniques. CAV is thought to be a chronic form of rejection, and evidence suggests that it might be related to recurrent episodes of acute cellular rejection, antibody mediated rejection, CMV infection, or other yet unrecognized factors.

Table 25.1	Cardiac Rejection Grading (ISHLT Scale, revised 2005).[5]
Grade 0R	No rejection
Grade 1R	Mild, low-grade, acute cellular rejection (previously 1A, 1B, and 2)— Interstitial and/or perivascular infiltrate with up to 1 focus of myocyte damage.
Grade 2R	Moderate, intermediate-grade, acute cellular rejection (previously 3A)—Two or more foci of infiltrate with associated myocyte damage.
Grade 3R	Severe, high-grade, acute cellular rejection (previously 3B and 4)—Diffuse infiltrate with multifocal myocyte damage ± edema ± hemorrhage ± vasculititis.

Additional Information:

AMR 0	Negative for AMR—No histological or immunopathologic features of AMR.
AMR 1	Positive for antibody-mediated rejection—Histologic features of AMR, positive immunoflourescence or immunoperoxidase staining for AMR (positive CD68, C4d)

AMR, antibody-mediated rejection

MEDICAL MANAGEMENT

Mild (ISHLT Grade 1R) cell mediated rejection: The intensity of treatment is variable and clinical judgment is necessary. For some asymptomatic patients with a grade 1R, adjustment of their current antirejection regimen is all that is necessary. In the patient with optimal immunosuppressant levels, especially in patients in the first 6 months posttransplantation, a 3-day course of 100 mg daily of prednisone along with repeat biopsy in 2 to 4 weeks can be considered. However, those with prominent symptoms early posttransplant period or with persistent abnormal biopsies should be hospitalized and treated with intravenous methylprednisolone 1000 mg daily for 3 days. The risk of progression from mild (ISHLT Grade 1R) is approximately 25% in the first 6 months posttransplant but becomes negligible after the first year.

Moderate (ISHLT Grade 2R) cell mediated rejection: As in all cases, the antirejection regimen should be optimized. In addition, therapy to resolve the acute rejection episode should be instituted (such as 3 days of 1000 mg intravenous methylprednisolone) along with repeat biopsy in 1 to 2 weeks to ensure resolution of the rejection.

Severe (ISHLT Grade 3R) cell mediated rejection: These patients should be evaluated for evidence of graft dysfunction. Intravenous methylprednisolone 1,000 mg daily should be instituted promptly and consideration given to additional immunosuppressive modalities. Additional options include cytolytic therapy with antithymocyte globulin or OKT3.

Rejection with hemodynamic compromise or antibody mediated rejection (AMR): All of these patients should be monitored in an intensive care unit with invasive hemodynamics and inotropic support as needed. Treatment consists of intravenous methylprednisone (as just noted) along with consideration for cytolytic therapy. Most patients (especially those with histologic evidence of AMR) should receive plasmapheresis. Weekly surveillance biopsies are indicated to ensure resolution of the rejection. Systemic anticoagulation with heparin should be considered given the tendency toward microvascular thrombosis.

CLINICAL PRESENTATION TIPS

- Asymptomatic: most cases of cell mediated rejection are asymptomatic and are detected on the basis of routine surveillance biopsies (Table 25.1).
- Contitutional Symptoms: should raise suspicion for rejection or occult infection
- Conduction abnormalities (atrial or ventricular arrhythmias, heart block, bundle branch block, sinus node dysfunction, etc): may be an early sign of graft irritability
- Heart Failure: suggests possible cell mediated and/or antibody mediated rejection and often needs invasive hemodynamic monitoring.

COMPLICATIONS

Renal failure is common in patients with severe heart failure and may be exacerbated posttransplant due to immunosuppressive agents—check the drug levels to ensure proper dosing.

CMV infection may present as fevers and constitutional symptoms or with pneumonia, gastritis, retinitis, or decreased white blood cell counts often in the context of treating acute graft rejection. Intravenous ganciclovir is often used to initiate therapy and an infectious disease consult should be considered.

Pneumocystis carinii pneumonia may also occur with increased immunosuppression in patients with graft rejection. Prophylaxis with trimethoprim-sulfamethoxazole should be utilized.

Neoplastic diseases may manifest in immunosuppressed patients.

CONCLUSIONS

Cardiac transplant patients require meticulous attention to histories and physicals, routine surveillance endomyocardial biopsies, and a high index of suspicion for cardiac allograft rejection. Prompt identification and treatment of rejection is important for prognosis and long-term outcome. Cardiac transplant patients presenting with hemodynamic compromise represent a high-risk group for whom immediate institution of antirejection measures should be utilized.

RECOMMENDED READING

1. Taylor DO, Edwards LB, Boucek MM, et al. Registry of the International Society for Heart and Lung Transplantation: twenty-second official adult heart transplant report—2005. *J Heart Lung Transplant.* 2005; 24:945–955.
2. Bourge RC, Rodriguez ER, Tan CD. Cardiac allograft rejection. In: Kirklin JK YJ, McGiffin DC, eds. *Heart Transplantation.* New York: Churchill Livingstone; 2002:464–520.
3. Lindenfeld J, Miller GG, Shakar SF, et al. Drug therapy in the heart transplant recipient: part I: cardiac rejection and immunosuppressive drugs. *Circulation.* 2004; 110:3734–3740.
4. Reed EF, Demetris AJ, Hammond E, et al. Acute antibody-mediated rejection of cardiac transplants. *J Heart Lung Transplant.* 2006; 25:153–159.
5. Stewart S, Winters GL, Fishbein MC, et al. Revision of the 1990 working formulation for the standardization of nomenclature in the diagnosis of heart rejection. *J Heart Lung Transplant.* 2005; 24:1710–1720.
6. Page RL, 2nd, Miller GG, Lindenfeld J. Drug therapy in the heart transplant recipient: part IV: drug-drug interactions. *Circulation.* 2005; 111:230–239.
7. Lindenfeld J, Page RL, 2nd, Zolty R, et al. Drug therapy in the heart transplant recipient: Part III: common medical problems. *Circulation.* 2005; 111:113–117.
8. Lindenfeld J, Miller GG, Shakar SF, et al. Drug therapy in the heart transplant recipient: part II: immunosuppressive drugs. *Circulation.* 2004; 110:3858–3865.

Procedures

CHAPTER 26

Right-Heart Catheterization

THOMAS H. WANG

INDICATIONS

- To differentiate between cardiogenic, septic, or hypovolemic shock
- Acute myocardial infarction (MI)
- Severe left-ventricular (LV) failure
- Cardiac tamponade
- To define the volume status and LV filling pressures

CONTRAINDICATIONS

- Coagulopathy
- INR >1.8
- Platelets <20,000
- Left bundle branch block is a relative contraindication due to the potential for complete heart block

DATA INTERPRETATION

A PA catheter can provide essential information in patients with severe cardiovascular disease. The data must be interpreted carefully in order to provide the most effective therapeutic intervention. In a hypotensive patient, the first step is to define whether the hypotension is due to a cardiogenic, hypovolemic, or septic etiology as indicated in Table 26.1.

The PA catheter can also be especially useful to define a specific clinical entity depending on a patient's presentation and the data available. Table 26.2 can help take the data seen on a PA catheter and help diagnose the disease.

ACUTE MANAGEMENT

Equipment:

- Ensure IV access, cardiac monitoring, an active type and screen, ECG, fluoroscopy (if available), cordis kit, and Swan-Ganz catheter; additionally, ultrasound guidance is advised if available

Procedure setup:

- Preferred site is the right internal jugular vein as it can be compressed if necessary, followed by left subclavian vein, followed by left internal jugular vein
- Femoral venous access may also be utilized but is technically more challenging and is associated with a greater risk of infection
- Left subclavian access may be considered but is less desirable due to the inability to compress the site should a hematoma occur

Post-procedure tests:

- CXR to rule out pneumothorax to confirm the PA catheter location

CCU Tip: Avoid left or right subclavian approach since many cardiac patients require a permanent pacemaker, an ICD, or BIV and a Swan-Ganz catheter in this location may distort the anatomy

Table 26.1	Differential of Shock.		
Data		Diagnosis	
Cardiac Output	PCWP	SVR	
Low	High	High	Cardiogenic
Low	Low	High	Hypovolemic
High	Low	Low	Septic

PCWP, pulmonary capillary wedge pressure; SVR, systemic vascular resistence

Table 26.2	Hemodynamic Findings

Data	Diagnosis
↑SvO$_2$ ↓BP O2 "step-up" of >5%	Acute VSD
RA mean = RVEDP = PCWP Pulsus paradoxicus Blunted y descent and prominent X descent on the RA tracing	Cardiac Tamponade
↑PCWP; suddenly prominent V wave on the PA wave tracing	Acute Mitral Regurgitation
↓CO ↓BP ↓RA CVP or RA pressure >PCWP Steep y descent on the RA tracing Right-sided ECG with ST elevation in V4	RV infarction
↑RA ↑PCWP Dip and plateau in the RV tracing M or W shaped JVP	Constriction
Normal PCWP but ↑PA ↑RV ↑RA	Pulmonary Embolism

BP, blood pressure; RA, right atrium; RVEDP, right-ventricle end diastolic pressure; PCWP, pulmonary capillary wedge pressure; PA, pulmonary artery; CO, cardiac output; CVP, central venous pressure; JVP, jugular venous pressure

LIMITATIONS OF DATA INTERPRETATION

While the PA catheter is incredibly useful, there are specific situations which limit the data that is provided. The pulmonary capillary wedge pressure (PCWP) is a useful monitor of LV filling pressure except in mitral stenosis, left-atrial myxoma, mitral regurgitation, acute aortic insufficiency, or in respiratory failure with high positive end expiratory pressure. With mitral stenosis, left-atrial myxoma or mitral regurgitation, the PCWP will tend to be erroneously high as left-atrial pressure is elevated over LV end diastolic pressure. With acute aortic insufficiency and high positive end expiratory pressures, the LV end diastolic pressure is greater than the left-atrial pressure, so the PCWP is erroneously low.

Limitations of the PA Catheter

Clinical Situation	Data Adjustment
Mitral Stenosis, Left-Atrial Myxoma, Mitral Regurgitation	Pulmonary capillary wedge pressure is erroneously high
Acute AI and high PEEP	Pulmonary capillary wedge pressure is erroneously low
Atrial Fibrillation/Flutter	
Severe Tricuspid Regurgitation	Thermodilution method is not
Low-Cardiac Output	reliable—use the Fick to
Intracardiac Shunt	calculate cardiac output.

The thermodilution method involves injecting saline into a proximal port and measuring the temperature change of the solution distally. It is not reliable in patients with an irregular heart rate, severe tricuspid regurgitation, an intracardiac shunt, and in low-cardiac output states because of the variability in blood flow. It is more reliable in a high-output state such as septic shock. The Fick method requires simultaneous measurement of the O_2 saturation from an arterial site and from the pulmonary artery. It is more accurate for an irregular rhythm and low-output states but cannot detect rapid changes in cardiac output.

Intracardiac Shunts
The PA catheter is especially useful in detecting intracardiac shunts. Under fluoroscopic guidance, blood may be sampled from the pulmonary artery (PA), the right ventricle (RV), the right atrium (RA), the inferior vena cava (IVC), and the superior vena cava (SVC). If fluoroscopy is not

COMPLICATIONS

- Respiratory distress and hypoxia may suggest a pneumothorax or hemothorax or pulmonary hemorrahge. Additionally, pulmonary artery rupture should be considered along with worsening valvular regurgitation due to catheter trauma.
- Arrhythmias can be due to irritation of the right ventricle and the right bundle.
- Hypotension can be due to blood loss due to an arterial rupture or a sepsis as the result of infection.
- Decreased platelets may suggest heparin induced thrombocytopenia.

available, then blood can be simply sampled from the PA and the RA (i.e., a distal and a proximal site). A "step up" or increase of O_2 saturation from a distal site compared to a proximal site indicates an intracardiac shunt. A step up of $\geq 7\%$ indicates an atrial shunt or $\geq 5\%$ indicates a shunt in the ventricle or at the PA level.

Complications

- **Pneumothorax/hemothorax:** generally caused due to erroneous placement of the introducer or needle. They can be minimized via the use of ultrasound guidance and easily diagnosed with a CXR.
- **Arterial laceration:** is also due to erroneous placement of the needle of introducer. Once again, ultrasound guidance can minimize this complication.
- **Complete heart block:** results from catheter irritation of the right bundle branch in a patient with pre-existing left bundle branch block. In this population, transcutaneous pacing should be readily available.
- **Pulmonary artery rupture:** occurs due to overwedging or overinflating the PA catheter in patients with elevated pulmonary pressures.
- **Tricuspid valvular trauma:** can occur when the catheter is withdrawn through the tricuspid valve when the balloon is inflated. Care should be taken to ensure that the balloon is deflated whenever withdrawing the catheter.
- **Heparin induced thrombocytopenia:** must be considered in patients with decreasing platelets without any source of heparin except the catheter. A nonheparin coated catheter may be utilized in these cases.
- **Sepsis:** strict sterile technique should be utilized with the insertion of a PA catheter. The introducer site should be regularly monitored for signs of infection.

RECOMMENDED READING

1. Cho L. Right heart catheterization. In: Griffin BP, Topol EJ, eds. *Manual of Cardiovascular Medicine.* 2nd ed. Philadelphia: Lippincott Williams & Wilkins; 2004:693–705.
2. Kern MJ, Feldman T, Bitar S. Hemodynamic data. In: *The Cardiac Catheterization Handbook.* 4th ed. St. Louis: Mosby; 2003:129–134.

CHAPTER 27

Temporary Transvenous Pacing

MEHDI H. SHISHEHBOR

INDICATIONS

Acute Myocardial Infarction

- New left bundle branch block with first-degree atrioventricular (AV) block
- Alternating right and left bundle branch block
- Mobitz type II block
- Complete heart block
- New right bundle branch block with either left anterior hemiblock or left posterior hemiblock

Right Ventricular Infarction

- Patients with loss of AV synchrony will need AV sequential pacing

Hemodynamically Significant Bradycardia

- Must correct underlying causes (i.e., digoxin toxicity)

Ventricular Tachycardia

- In patients with long QT syndrome
- Bradycardia-dependent ventricular tachycardia

Hemodynamically Significant Chronotropic Incompetence

- Aortic insufficiency
- Severe heart failure
- Bridge to permanent pacing

ACUTE MANAGEMENT

Preparation

Informed consent

Equipment:

- Two large-bore IV lines, cardiac monitor, cardiopulmonary resuscitation equipment, fluoroscopy.

Procedure setup:

- Preferred site is right internal jugular vein
- May also use left subclavian if permanent pacemaker (PPM) not planned
- Occasionally femoral vein can be used however this position is the least stable
- Before becoming sterile patient should be placed in appropriate position and drapped in sterile fashion

Post-procedure tests:

- Chest x-ray to rule out pneumothorax, confirm pacer wire location
- ECG-Should have a left bundle branch block pattern with left axis deviation

Pacer Care:

- Daily ECG
- Determine daily pacing and sensing thresholds
- Determine intrinsic rhythm when indicated
- Check insertion site for sign of infection and apply daily dressing

CONTRAINDICATION

Coagulopathy
- INR >1.8
- Platelet <50,000

PLACEMENT

- Position and drape patient as above.
- After local anesthetic, insert a 5F venous sheath.

- Under fluoroscopy, advance pacing wire.
- Use clockwise and/or counter-clockwise rotation to cross the tricuspid valve.
- Avoid using excessive force.
- Once inside the right ventricle (RV), the catheter tip should point inferiorly.
- Mild amount of bulking in systole is acceptable.
- However, excessive bulking may cause perforation.
- Avoid placing the pacing wire in the true apex, the ideal position is the diaphragmatic wall of RV between middle to apical segment.
- Pacing at other locations may be possible, but it is frequently associated with pacer wire dislodgement.
- For right-atrial (RA) pacing, a second 5F venous sheath is needed
- Use a 5F J-tiped pacing wire.
- The ideal position is a J-shape figure from the LAO view or an L-shape figure from the RAO view.

PACER THRESHOLD TESTING

Capture Threshold
- This is measured in mA.
- Begin pacing at a rate of 10 to 15 beats over the intrinsic rate.
- Starting output is usually set at 5 mA.
- If no capture at this output, reposition pacer wire.
- If capture present, then slowly decrease until capture is lost.
- The lowest capturing current is pacing threshold.
- Set pacing output three times the pacing threshold (minimum 3 mA).

Sensing Threshold
- This is measured in mV.
- Gradually decrease sensing threshold until asynchronous pacing is seen.
- This is sensing threshold.
- Set pacer at twice the sensing threshold.

Atrioventricular Delay
- This is used for dual chamber pacing.
- The default is usually at 150 msec.
- Must be tailored to patient's condition (i.e., if need longer diastolic filling time then AV delay should be longer) may use hemodynamic numbers to guide AV delay time.

COMPLICATIONS

- Hypotension: suspect pneumothorax, hemothorax, myocardial perforation and tamponade, dyssynchrony secondary to right-ventricule pacing
- Hypoxia: suspect pneumothorax, hemothorax, or air embolus
- Arrhythmias: pacer position
- Decreased urine output: hemothorax, myocardial perforation, tamponade, worsening heart failure secondary to dyssynchronoy
- Complete heart block: in setting of left bundle branch block due to irritation of right bundle, usually transient in nature
- Pacer dysfunction: electrode dislodgement, over or undersensing, generator failure
- Infection: time interval since insertion

COMPLICATIONS

- **Pericardial effusion/tamponade:** Aggressive volume resuscitation and pericardiocentesis if hemodynamic compromise (i.e., tamponade).
- **Hemothorax:** Volume and blood resuscitation, chest tube insertion, immediate cardiothoracic consultation.
- **Dyssynchrony:** May need BiV pacing.
- **Complete heart block:** In patients with left branch bundle block (LBBB) secondary to irritation of right bundle. Usually transient in nature.
- **Pneumothorax:** If significant usually >25% to 30% will need chest tube, if <20% and patient hemodynamically stable may monitor in the cardiac intensive care unit (CICU) with serial chest x-rays.

RECOMMENDED READING

1. Kern MJ, Bitar S, Puri S. Special techniques. In: Kern, MJ, ed. *The Cardiac Catheterization Handbook.* St. Louis: Mosby-Year Book; 1991:309–313.
2. Mukherjee D. Temporary transvenous pacing. In: Griffin BP, and Topol EJ, ed. *Manual of Cardiovascular Medicine.* Philadelphia: Lippincott Williams & Wilkins; 2004:706–708.

CHAPTER 28

Pericardiocentesis

THOMAS H. WANG

INDICATIONS

Cardiac Tamponade

- A clinical diagnosis with hypotension, tachycardia, and jugular venous distention (JVD).
- Echocardiographic signs with diastolic right-ventricular (RV) and systolic right-atrial (RA) collapse, mitral and tricuspid valve respiratory variation, inferior and vena cava (IVC) plethora (Chapter 18).

CONTRAINDICATIONS

- Left-ventricular (LV) free-wall rupture
- Type-A dissection
- Posterior effusion
- Recurrent malignant effusions
- Coagulopathy
- INR >1.8
- Platelets <50,000

PLACEMENT

- Position and drape patient.
- Confirm apical, parasternal, or subcostal approach with echocardiography.
- Mark the skin at the echo transducer site.
- Sterilize the field.
- Anesthetize the access point with lidocaine; ensure a track that proceeds over a rib.

A C U T E M A N A G E M E N T

Preparation

Informed consent

Equipment:

- Two large-bore IV lines, cardiac monitor, cardiopulmonary resuscitation equipment

Procedure setup:

- Make sure patient has at least two large-bore IV access sites and an active type and screen.
- Use apical, parasternal, and subcostal approach depending on effusion size at each location.
- Mark entry site prior to sterilizing the field with echocardiographic guidance.
- Ensure that the angle of needle entry is parallel to the echo transducer angle and note the distance to the effusion.

Postprocedure tests:

- Use Echo to reevaluate effusion size and to inject agitated saline to define catheter location.
- Use CXR to assess for a pneumothorax.
- Catheter drain care—the catheter should be aspirated every 6 hours followed by a sterile saline flush; monitor the catheter site for signs of infection. The drain may be discontinued when the drainage is less than 50 cc/day.
- Avoid leaving the catheter in place for longer than 24 hours.

CCU Tip: Consider placing an 8F cordis for venous access in case of emergency—if the position of the needle or catheter tip is in doubt, inject agitated saline; do not remove the catheter if it is located in the right ventricle.

- Confirm needle angle with echo transducer and distance to the effusion.
- Insert needle until fluid return is detected; typically this occurs after a gentle "pop" is felt.
- Confirm needle location with agitated saline injection under echo guidance.

- Advance a wire through the needle and withdraw the needle.
- Insert the catheter over the wire—reconfirm position with agitated saline.

CONFIRMATORY STUDIES

Agitated Saline
- Inject agitated saline via a 3-way stopcock.
- Bubbles within a cardiac chamber suggest perforation.

Bloody Fluid
- Inject a bloody aspirate onto a clean gauze.
- Blood clot suggests chamber perforation; pericardial effusions that are bloody typically do not clot.

Clinical Response:
- Rapid and dramatic improvement in hemodynamics—an immediate decrease in heart rate and increase in blood pressure may be seen.

LABORATORY STUDIES

- Assess for infectious etiology.
- Send for bacterial and viral cultures as well as cytomegalovirus (CMV) and cocksackie virus cultures.
- If mycobacterium suspected, check acid-fast bacillus smear and culture.
- Assess for malignancy.
- Cell count and cytology.
- Assess for rheumatic origin.
- Antinuclear antibody and rheumatoid factor.

COMPLICATIONS

- Hypotension: suspect pneumothorax, hemothorax, myocardial perforation; also consider an arterial laceration if the needle puncture site is below the rib or if an anterior or subxiphoid approach is taken, which can jeopardize the left internal mammary artery.
- Hypoxia: suspect pneumothorax or hemothorax.
- Arrhythmias: consider right-ventricular irritation, right-ventricular perforation, left-ventricular irritation or perforation.

COMPLICATIONS

- **Hemothorax:** Volume and blood resuscitation, chest tube insertion, immediate cardiothoracic consultation.
- **Pneumothorax:** If significant usually >25% to 30% will need chest tube; if <20% and patient hemodynamically stable, may monitor in the coronary care unit (CICU) with serial chest x-rays.
- **Myocardial Perforation:** Leave the catheter in place—do not attempt to remove the catheter. Immediate cardiothoracic consultation.
- **Infection:** Use sterile technique during preparation and consider antibiotic therapy if access site or catheter appears infected.
- **Arterial laceration:** Follow with frequent hematocrit checks and blood transfusions as necessary. May need a surgical consult.

RECOMMENDED READING

1. Kern MJ, Bitar S, Puri S. Special techniques. In: Kern MJ, ed. *The Cardiac Catheterization Handbook.* St. Louis: Mosby-Year Book; 2003:309–313.
2. Gring C, Griffin BP. Pericardiocentesis. In: Griffin BP, Topol EJ, ed. *Manual of Cardiovascular Medicine.* Philadelphia: Lippincott Williams & Wilkins; 2004:709–713.

CHAPTER 29

Cardioversion

TIMOTHY H. MAHONEY

INDICATIONS

I. Emergent/Immediate
   A. Ventricular fibrillation (VF)
   B. Hemodynamically unstable ventricle tachycardia (VT)
   C. Hemodynamically unstable superventricular tachycardia (SVT)
   D. Atrial fibrillation (AF) in the following settings:
      1. Hypotension
      2. Atrial fibrillation with evidence of acute myocardial infarction (MI)
      3. Atrial fibrillation with evidence of acute heart failure that does not respond to medical management.
      4. Atrial fibrillation with angina despite medical therapy
II. Elective
   A. Hemodynamically stable VT
   B. Atrial fibrillation/flutter of <48 hours or >48 hours if INR >2.0 for 3 weeks or a negative TEE.
   C. Hemodynamically stable SVT

CONTRAINDICATIONS

- Hemodynamically stable chronic AF not on anticoagulation
- An improperly sedated patient
- Sinus rhythm/sinus tachycardia

PREPARATION & EQUIPMENT

A. For elective cardioversion, patient should be nothing by mouth (NPO)

B. Oxygen should be delivered via face mask

C. Anesthesia: For elective/urgent cardioversion in hemodynamically stable individuals, conscious sedation should be used

D. Electrode placement

  1. Sternal-apex or anterior-apex approach: provides lower energy

    a. Sternal or anterior electrode placed on the right side of the sternum below the clavicle.

    b. Apical electrode should be placed left of the nipple in the midaxillary line.

  2. Anterior posterior placement:

    a. Anterior paddle should be placed at apex as in sternal-apex approach.

    b. Posterior paddle should be placed in the left infrascapular area.

    c. Special considerations

      i. Permanent pacemaker (PPM): Avoid contact with device. Keep paddle at least 1 inch away. Postshock device should be interrogated to ensure proper function.

      ii. Defibrillator: Same rules of positioning and interrogation as PPM. Allow 60 seconds post-ICD shock to reassess rhythm if device fires during code.

    d. Transcutaneous pacer available given risk of asystole or symptomatic bradycardia after successful defibrillation/cardioversion.

    e. Anticoagulation in setting of hemodynamically stable atrial fibrillation (AF) lasting more than 48 hours.

  1. Anticoagulate 3 to 4 weeks prior and 4 weeks postcardioversion to normal sinus rhythm.

  2. If TEE performed to rule out LAA thrombus, anticoagulate at time of cardioversion and for at least 4 weeks after.

BASIC PRINCIPLES/DEFINITIONS

I. Ohm's Law: Current = Voltage/Impedance

II. Impedance: A measure of resistance across the path on which energy is delivered.

  A. Decreasing impedance increases current delivered.

  B. Besides amount of energy delivered, medical personnel can affect current delivery by regulating impedance. Impedance can be affected by the following:

1. Electrode Size: Larger, the lower the impedance.
2. Placement: In women, avoiding breast tissue will decrease impedance.
3. Contact to skin: Maintaining firm contact with pads decreases impedance.
4. Shock timing: Impedance decreases with number of shocks and decreased time between shocks.
5. Respiratory cycle: Impedance lowest at end expiration.

MODES

A. Precordial Thump: Use controversial. Success rates estimated to be 11% to 25% for termination of ventricular tachycardia (VT). Success rates much lower for VF.
B. Electrical
   1. Synchronized: Mode used to ensure no impulse delivered during cardiac vulnerable period. Vulnerable period includes the 60 to 80 msec prior and 20 to 30 msec after the apex of the T wave. Prevents induction of VF by shock. Used for supraventricular tachycardia (SVT), AF, atrial flutter (Aflutter), and hemodynamically stable wide complex tachycardia (WCT).
   2. Unsynchronized: Reserved for VF and polymorphic VT.
   3. Monophasic: Traditional method of energy delivery. Current delivered in one direction.
   4. Biphasic: Current flows in one direction for a period of time and then reverses direction. Thus, passes through area of shock delivery twice.
      a. Requires less energy delivery.
      b. Little data supporting superior maintenance of sinus rhythm over long term.
      c. Some data it may be more successful in cardioverting AF.

Defibrillation: Term used for the delivery of energy to terminate VF and polymorphic VT. The following is a list of suggested energy delivery for monophasic defibrillator.

- Unsynchronized
- First Shock: 200J
- Second shock: 200 to 300J
- Third and subsequent shocks: 360J

Cardioversion: Term used for delivery of energy to terminate SVT, AF, Aflutter, and hemodynamically stable VT. The following are recommend monophasic shock energy.

- Aflutter, AF, or SVT: Note Aflutter and SVT may respond to 50J shock. Subsequent shocks 100, 200, 300, and then 360J.
- Stable/monomorphic ventricular tachycardia: 100, 200, 300, and then 360J.

COMPLICATIONS

- Embolism in setting of chronic atrial fibrillation not anticoagulated, risk 1% to 7%.
- Arrhythmias
  - VT/VF: increased likelihood in digitalis toxic patients and electrolyte abnormalities
  - Asystole
  - Bradycardia
- Mild elevation in cardiac enzymes.
- Atrial dysfunction/standstill may occur in postcardioversion of atrial fibrillation.
- Pulmonary edema likely due to atrial dysfunction.
- Skin burns occur in up to 25% of all patients.

RECOMMENDED READING

1. Gurm HS, Schweikert RA. Electrical cardioversion. In: Griffin BP, Topol EJ, ed. *Manual of Cardiovascular Medicine.* Philadelphia: Lippincott Williams & Wilkins; 2004:714–719.
2. American Heart Association. *Automated External Defibrillation. ACLS: Principles and Practice.*

CHAPTER 30

Intra-aortic Balloon Counterpulsation

TARAL N. PATEL

Inta-aortic balloon counterpulsation or pumping (IABP) is the most commonly used circulatory assist device with over 70,000 procedures yearly in the United States alone. IABP assists and augments left-ventricular (LV) function through inflation and deflation of a balloon catheter inserted into the descending aorta and timed to the cardiac cycle. Indications for use of IABP include hemodynamic circulatory support in acute unstable settings and to provide a bridge to definitive therapy. Additionally, technological advances in catheter size and insertion techniques have decreased complications considerably.

INDICATIONS

- Refractory cardiogenic shock due to
  - Myocardial infarction (MI)
  - Mechanical complications of acute MI such as papillary muscle rupture or ventricular-septal defect
  - Severe acute mitral regurgitation due to endocarditis or leaflet tear/ flail
  - Acute myocarditis
  - End-stage cardiomyopathy—bridge to definitive therapy
  - Severe myocardial contusion
- Unstable angina refractory to medical therapy
- Ischemic ventricular tachyarrhythmias refractory to medical therapy
- Adjunctive therapy during high-risk percutaneous coronary intervention (PCI) or primary PCI for acute MI

- Prophylaxis for severe left main coronary artery disease awaiting surgery
- Failure to wean from cardiopulmonary bypass
- Decompensated severe aortic stenosis awaiting definitive therapy

CONTRAINDICATIONS

Absolute
- Severe aortic insufficiency
- Aortic dissection/aneurysm
- Patent ductus arteriosus

Relative
- Moderate aortic insufficiency
- Severe peripheral vascular disease:
  - Previous descending/peripheral arterial surgery such as femoral-popliteal bypass grafting
- Sepsis
- Acute or previous bleeding diathesis
- Contraindication to use of intravenous anticoagulation

PHYSIOLOGY AND HEMODYNAMICS

The principle hemodynamic benefits of IABP are achieved through reduction of cardiac afterload, augmentation of diastolic coronary artery perfusion, and reduction of myocardial oxygen demand. During systole there is rapid balloon deflation resulting in a vacuum-like effect in the aorta. Thus, aortic end diastolic pressure and systolic blood pressure are decreased below baseline, which leads to a salutary decrease in ventricular wall stress and myocardial oxygen consumption. During diastole there is rapid balloon inflation resulting in an increase in diastolic blood pressure above systolic level in many patients. Overall direct and indirect effects of IABP support result in

- 20% decrease in systolic blood pressure
- 30% increase in diastolic blood pressure
- reduction of heart rate by <20%
- 20% decrease in pulmonary capillary wedge pressure (PCWP)
- 20% increase in cardiac output
- 14% decrease in LV wall stress

Displacement of blood to the proximal and distal aorta in diastole also theoretically results in improved organ, tissue, and coronary perfusion although this last point is controversial. Hemodynamic studies have demonstrated increased flow in the proximal coronary arteries and proximal to a severe stenosis in a given diseased vessel, but no increase in poststenotic flow. Further, there is no augmentation in collateral coronary flow. Therefore, reductions in LV wall stress and myocardial oxygen demand seem paramount in explaining the benefits of IABP support.

PROCEDURE

- **Patient preparation:** A detailed discussion of the risks, benefits, and alternatives to the procedure and the limited mobility of the patient during therapy should be undertaken whenever possible. The appropriate groin should be sterilely prepared to the knee, draped, and local anesthetic should be infiltrated in the skin where the sheath is to be inserted.
- **Anatomy:** Percutaneous insertion of the IABP is usually accomplished through the common femoral artery, below the inguinal ligament. Prior to the procedure, femoral and distal pulses should be palpated on both sides. If there is a suspicion for peripheral vascular disease (PVD), the side with the strongest pulse or highest ankle/brachial index should be utilized.
- **Sizing and preparation of balloon:** Balloon volumes vary and choice of appropriate balloon size is based on the height of the patient (Table 30.1). The one-way valve at the proximal end of the catheter is first to be attached to the male leuer fitting of the extracorporeal tubing. A

Table 30.1	Balloon membrane dimensions and sizing chart.				
Balloon Membrane Volume (cc)	Balloon Membrane Dimensions			Patient Height	
	Length (mm)	Diameter (mm)	(ft)	(cm)
25	174	14.7	<5′	<152
34	219	14.7	5′0″–5′4″	152–162
40	263	15	5′4″–6′0″	162–183
50	269	16.3	>6′0″	>183

Adapted from Datascope® Corporation with permission.

60 cc syringe is then attached to the other end of the one-way valve and negative suction applied to withdraw excess air from the balloon and ease insertion. The stylet wire is removed from the inner lumen of the catheter and the inner lumen is flushed with saline.

- **Access and insertion:** Access to the common femoral artery is commonly obtained using an 18-gauge introducer needle. A J-tipped guidewire (provided in the IABP kit) is advanced through the needle to the arch of the aorta. Guidewire and subsequent balloon advancement should be undertaken with fluoroscopic guidance. After access is secured and the guidewire is in place, the femoral arteriotomy site is enlarged with a vessel dilator to facilitate insertion of the sheath (8 to 10.5 French). Typically, a second dilator is inserted into the sheath, and the entire system flushed with saline and inserted into the femoral artery over the guidewire. The dilator is then removed with the sheath and the guidewire left in place. The end of the guidewire is subsequently inserted into the distal end of the inner lumen and advanced until it exits the female leuer hub of the balloon. With the guidewire fixed, the tip of the IABP is advanced to the descending aorta, just below the left subclavian artery. Using fluoroscopy, the tracheal carina can be used as an appropriate landmark to indicate the appropriate position of the balloon tip. The guidewire and one-way valve with gas-lumen insert are removed and blood aspirated from the inner lumen. Standard arterial pressure monitoring tubing is attached to the inner lumen and gas tubing is attached to the male leuer fitting. The sheath seal is then advanced to the sheath to cover the length of exposed catheter outside of the body. Finally, the balloon is filled with helium gas and pumping is initiated, preferably under fluoroscopic monitoring during initial balloon inflation to ensure proper deployment. The position of the balloon is verified again prior to securing the catheter to the leg with suture.
- **Anticoagulation:** Intravenous heparin is typically administered to maintain the activated partial thromboplastin time (aPTT) at 50 to 70 seconds.
- **Post-IABP care:** Patients undergoing IABP therapy must lie supine for the duration of support. Excessive limb movement can result in significant bleeding and even femoral artery laceration; therefore adequate sedation and analgesia are necessary to allow the patient to remain still. Lower extremities should be examined and distal arterial pulses palpated frequently to check for signs of limb ischemia. Daily chest x-rays should be obtained to check IABP position.

SPECIAL CIRCUMSTANCES

- **Insertion without the use of fluoroscopy:** If fluoroscopy is not available for IABP insertion, the distance from the sternal angle of Louis to the umbilicus and then to the femoral arterial puncture site is measured. The IABP is then inserted to this distance and can be used while a chest x-ray is immediately obtained to check position and make adjustments. To make adjustments to catheter position, the IABP is placed on standby while the catheter is either withdrawn or advanced to the proper position and resecured.

- **Sheathless insertion:** The IABP can be inserted directly into the femoral artery and aorta without a sheath over the guidewire. This technique may reduce complications of lower-limb ischemia in patients with PVD. However, once placed, the IABP cannot be readily adjusted without contamination and there is a higher risk of infection when placing the catheter without a sheath.

- **Surgical insertion:** If percutaneous access cannot be obtained, the IABP can be inserted surgically using a cutdown to expose the femoral artery. The catheter can then be inserted via direct arteriotomy or into a prosthetic conduit that is anastomosed to the femoral artery in an end-to-side fashion. These methods may reduce the risk of limb ischemia; however, when therapy is discontinued, the IABP has to be removed and the artery repaired surgically. Additionally, the IABP can be inserted surgically into the descending aorta via left subclavian artery cutdown in the setting of prohibitive bilateral lower-extremity PVD. This type of insertion is rare.

- **Contraindication to the use of anticoagulation:** Traditionally, IABP therapy has been contraindicated when anticoagulation cannot be administered to prevent thrombosis. However, a recent randomized trial demonstrated no major complications or thrombosis of the balloon catheter in 82 patients randomized to withholding of anticoagulation (Jiang et al.).

DISCONTINUATION OF IABP THERAPY

- **Weaning:** Typically, prior to withdrawal of the IABP, decreasing levels of support are attempted to ensure hemodynamic stability. Most commonly, a frequency weaning approach is used, where augmentation of every second beat (1:2), then every third (1:3) is undertaken for 1 to 2 hours each. A second, less frequently used method is to reduce balloon volume by increments of 20% in a step-wise fashion until the volume cycled is approximately 20% of the original. This volume weaning process may be more physiologic than frequency weaning, however, there may be greater risk of thrombus formation. During the weaning process blood pressure, heart rate, urine output and cardiac index and pulmonary capillary wedge pressure (if available) are closely monitored for signs of instability. Inotropic drugs or vasodilators can be introduced at this time if necessary to facilitate weaning and discontinue IABP support. If weaning is tolerated, augmentation is changed back to 1:1 or volume restored to 100% until the IABP can be discontinued.

- **Removal of catheter:** Anticoagulation should be discontinued at least 4 hours prior to actual removal of the IABP. An activated clotting time (ACT) or aPTT should be checked to ensure that anticoagulation has worn off adequately. After all sutures have been removed the IABP should be placed on standby and helium driveline disconnected. Holding pressure at the sheath site, the balloon catheter should be withdrawn until resistance is felt. This indicates that the proximal end of the balloon has reached the tip of the sheath. The sheath and catheter should then be grasped as a unit and removed from the femoral artery while firm pressure is applied just distal to the puncture site. The artery should be allowed bleed directly out of the leg for 1 to 2 pulsations to remove any thrombus that may have been lodged at the arteriotomy site from the balloon. Firm, nonocclusive pressure should then be applied just above the puncture site, for 25 to 35 minutes to achieve hemostasis.

- **Postremoval care:** Distal arterial pulses should be monitored during and for several hours after the removal of the catheter to assess for limb ischemia. Patients should be required to remain supine for a minimum of 6 hours after removal. A pressure dressing should be applied at the puncture site with hourly groin checks to assess for bleeding or hematoma formation. Anticoagulation for reasons other than IABP therapy alone can be restarted 6 hours after removal and hemostasis.

CHANGING THE IABP

- **Indications:** In the setting of prolonged IABP therapy, some centers recommend routine changing of the balloon catheter and sheath after a set period of time to prevent infectious complications. If iatrogenic infection is suspected but IABP therapy is still required, the balloon catheter and sheath should be changed. Additional reasons for changing the catheter and sheath include perforation of the balloon, kinking or other malfunction of the catheter resulting in inadequate balloon inflation, and balloon entrapment.

- **Techniques:** Typically, a fresh access site in the contralateral femoral artery is used when exchanging IABP catheters. Often, simultaneous exchange is required because the patient may be IABP "dependent." After access is obtained, a guidewire is advanced into the aorta with the old balloon on standby. The old IABP can then be turned on, while the new one is prepared and appropriate connections as made. The old IABP is then turned off and removed as just described, and the new IABP advanced to the appropriate position while pressure is held at the old site.

- If the contralateral femoral artery is not able to be utilized or accessed, the IABP catheter can be changed over a wire. This approach, however, is associated with a higher incidence of infection and should not be utilized if the indication for IABP exchange is fever. If this is the case, the IABP can be exchanged using a surgical cutdown technique while suturing the old arteriotomy site.

TIMING AND TRIGGERING

Ideal timing and triggering are essential for appropriate IABP function and maximal hemodynamic benefit to the patient. IABP inflation should occur on the downslope of the aortic pressure waveform just prior to the dicrotic notch (aortic valve closure), while deflation should occur at end diastole prior to the initiation of the next systolic pulse (Fig. 30.1). Though the timing of inflation and deflation can be adjusted manually, modern IABP consoles adjust these parameters automatically to maintain optimal performance. In order for proper timing to occur, a trigger for inflation and deflation must be selected. Typical triggers that are used include the ECG waveform and arterial pressure waveform. If the ECG is used, inflation should occur during the middle of the T wave, which corresponds to early ventricular diastole, and deflation should occur at the peak of the R wave corresponding to the beginning of systole (see Fig. 30.1).

- **Early inflation:** This occurs when the inflation of the IABP occurs well ahead of aortic valve closure. This may result in early valve closure, aortic regurgitation, decreased stroke volume, and increased LV wall stress, end-diastolic pressure, and myocardial oxygen demand (Fig. 30.2).

- **Late inflation:** This occurs when inflation occurs well after aortic valve closure. This may result in suboptimal diastolic augmentation and coronary artery perfusion (Fig. 30.3).

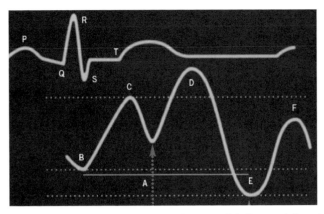

FIGURE 30.1. Proper timing of IABP inflation and deflation. Adapted from Datascope® Corporation with permission.

A = one complete cardiac cycle
B = unassisted aortic end diastolic pressure
C = unassisted aortic systolic pressure
D = diastolic augmentation
E = assisted aortic end diastolic pressure
F = assisted aortic systolic pressure

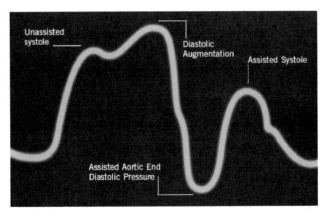

FIGURE 30.2. Early balloon inflation. Adapted from Datascope® Corporation with permission.

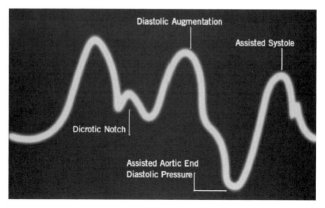

FIGURE 30.3. Late balloon inflation. Adapted from Datascope® Corporation with permission.

- **Early deflation:** This occurs when deflation occurs well prior to initiation of ventricular isovolumic contraction. This may result in suboptimal diastolic augmentation, coronary artery perfusion, and afterload reduction resulting in an increase in myocardial oxygen demand (Fig. 30.4).
- **Late deflation:** This occurs when deflation occurs after the onset of isovolumic contraction. This results in impaired ventricular emptying, increased afterload and preload, and reduced stroke volume resulting in increased myocardial oxygen demand (Fig. 30.5).

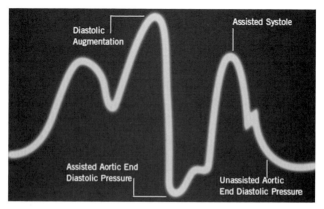

FIGURE 30.4. Early balloon deflation. Adapted from Datascope® Corporation with permission.

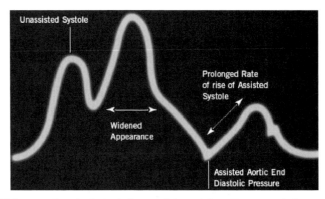

FIGURE 30.5. Late balloon deflation. Adapted from Datascope® Corporation with permission.

INAPPROPRIATE AUGMENTATION

Suboptimal hemodynamic benefit of the IABP may result from a combination of multiple mechanical issues and patient-related issues. Improper or loose connections, kinking of the IABP catheter resulting in impaired gas shuttling, or perforation or entrapment of the balloon can be assessed by checking the connections, looking for blood in the gas driveline, and visualizing the IABP under fluoroscopy. Impaired augmentation resulting from inappropriate triggering may result from noisy ECG leads or arrhythmias. In the case of noisy ECG leads, the leads can be changed or the trigger changed to the aortic pulse waveform. In the presence of tachyarrhythmias, adequate augmentation is often difficult or impossible to achieve. When the heart rate approaches 150 beats per minute, there is insufficient time for gas shuttling. The IABP may have to be switched to assist 1:2 to provide more reliable inflation and deflation. Treatment of the underlying arrhythmias, if possible, should obviously be undertaken. In the setting of sepsis, peripheral vasodilation may prevent proper IABP augmentation.

COMPLICATIONS

Although improvements in IABP technology and increased usage have dramatically reduced the invasiveness and complication rate of the procedure, there are well-known adverse effects that are critical to recognize. In the largest registry of IABP use, the overall complication rate was 7%, while major complications, such as limb ischemia and major bleeding occurred in 2.6% of patients. Several factors were associated with an increased risk of complications including age ≥75 years, PVD, diabetes mellitus, female gender, prolonged support, and small-body surface area.

COMPLICATIONS

- Access site bleeding: Bleeding may result from trauma or perforation of the femoral artery during insertion, excessive anticoagulation, or inadequate hemostasis after IABP removal. In most cases, manual pressure can be held at the sheath site while anticoagulation issues are corrected if present. Transfusion may be indicated for excessive blood loss. If bleeding is persistent or a pseudoaneurysm is suspected and diagnosed by ultrasound, thrombin injection or direct surgical repair of the arteriotomy may be indicated.

- Infection: As with any indwelling catheter, insertion of the IABP poses a risk of infection to the patient that increases with increasing duration of support. Some experts recommend immediate discontinuation of therapy in the presence of fever in a patient with no other obvious source of infection. It is our practice to discontinue therapy if no longer absolutely necessary. If infection is suspected, and support continues to be necessary, the balloon pump can be changed to the contralateral side through a new access site and intravenous antibiotics can be administered.

- Hemolysis and thrombocytopenia: Mechanical destruction of blood cells leading to a decrease in circulating red cells and platelets is commonly noted in patients treated with IABP. Therefore, daily complete blood counts should be obtained. The degree of hemolysis and thrombocytopenia appears to be related to the duration of therapy and the destruction subsides when therapy is discontinued. Though red blood cell transfusion may occasionally be required, thrombocytopenia below 50,000 is rare.

- Dissection: Aortic dissection typically occurs during insertion of the guidewire or balloon catheter. Operators must have a high level of suspicion for this complication if any amount of resistance to catheter insertion is felt. If dissection is suspected, particularly if the patient experiences back or abdominal pain, the procedure should be aborted, the catheter removed, and appropriate diagnostic studies obtained.

- Thromboembolism and organ ischemia: Thrombus is not uncommonly seen around the IABP catheter at the time of removal. Renal emboli, splenic infarction, mesenteric and spinal ischemia, and peripheral emboli have all been well described in the literature and vigilance is required in monitoring for these complications. Evidence of organ ischemia often necessitates discontinuation of therapy.

- Limb ischemia: Limb ischemia may result from thromboembolism, atheroembolism, arterial dissection, or insertion of a large catheter into a small and/or diseased femoral artery. Signs and symptoms of limb ischemia include a cold limb, loss of peripheral pulses, pain, paresthesias, and pallor, while levido reticularis and eosiniphilia are specific for

atheroembolism. Evidence of limb ischemia necessitates a switch to the contraleteral limb or discontinuation of therapy.
* Rupture, perforation, or entrapment of the balloon: Rupture or perforation of the IABP is rare but often catastrophic and is thought to be related to repetitive inflation against calcified plaque in the aorta. This can lead to gas embolism and/or thrombosis within the balloon and subsequent entrapment of the IABP in the aorta. The most common sign of perforation or rupture is the presence of blood within the gas lumen of the catheter. This complication requires immediate and often surgical removal of the catheter because of entrapment.

RECOMMENDED READING

1. Quaal, SJ. *Comprehensive Intraaortic Balloon Counterpulsation.* 2nd ed. St. Louis: Mosby; 1993.
2. Roe MT. Intraaortic balloon counterpulsation. In: Marso SP, Griffin BP, Topol EJ (eds.). *Manual of Cardiovascular Medicine.* Philadelphia: Lippincott Williams & Wilkins; 2000:687–699.
3. Laham RJ, Aroesty JM. Intraaortic balloon pump counterpulsation. In: UpToDateVersion14.2, 2006.
4. Trost JC, Hillis LD. Intra-aortic Balloon Counterpulsation. *Am J Cardiol.* 2006; 97:1391–1398.

Miscellaneous

CHAPTER 31

Ventilator Management in the Cardiac Care Unit

EDUARDO MIRELES-CABODEVILA

ALEJANDRO C. ARROLIGA

M echanical ventilation (MV) is often required to support patients with respiratory failure in the coronary care unit (CCU). Cardiovascular diseases account for 29% of the nonoperative causes of respiratory failure, with an associated mortality of 24% to 33%. Congestive heart failure (CHF) decreases lung compliance and increases alveolar edema, thus reducing ventilatory capacity and increasing the work of breathing. If untreated, this can be an unbearable burden for the ailing heart. Recognizing the effects of the positive pressure ventilation on the cardiovascular system helps in maximizing its benefits and minimizing its adverse effects.

EFFECTS OF MECHANICAL VENTILATION ON THE CARDIOVASCULAR SYSTEM

MV applies positive pressure both during inspiration and expiration. It decreases preload and afterload by increasing the intrathoracic pressure. Preload is reduced via decreased venous return whereas afterload is diminished via decreased left-ventricular (LV) transmural myocardial stress. In patients whose hemodynamic status depends on an adequate preload, MV may precipitate hemodynamic collapse and should be addressed with volume resuscitation.

Positive-end expiratory pressure (PEEP) also has significant hemodynamic effects, which are more evident with increased lung compliance. PEEP will improve V/Q matching and gas exchange by preventing alveolar collapse, increasing functional residual capacity, and redistributing fluid in the alveoli. This will manifest as increased blood oxygen and decreased ventilator-induced lung injury. However, it can also decrease preload and thus negatively affect cardiac output. PEEP is utilized with care in the CCU setting.

NONINVASIVE MECHANICAL VENTILATION (NIMV)

NIMV uses positive pressure to support ventilation and oxygenation via a tight seal mask. There are two types: continuous positive airway pressure (CPAP) and bilevel-positive airway pressure. NIMV should not be used in the case of a facial abnormality or lesion which prevents an adequate seal, inability to protect the airway, severe hypoxemia (i.e., FiO_2 100%), hemodynamic instability, significant arrhythmia, and acute intra-abdominal process (including upper gastrointestinal [GI] bleed).

Use of NIMV in the CCU

- CPAP and Bilevel positive airway pressure improve oxygenation and reduce the incidence of intubation in pulmonary edema.
- Bilevel positive airway pressure has been recommended when respiratory acidosis is present in addition to pulmonary edema.
- CPAP and Bilevel positive airway pressure reduce the rate of reintubation when used directly after extubation in patients at high risk of reintubation. It is not useful as a rescue therapy once patients have failed extubation.

Note: If a patient has not improved his or her parameters after 2 to 4 hours of NIMV, this mode is unlikely to avoid intubation.

COMPLICATIONS OF MECHANICAL VENTILATION

MV can cause an array of side effects and complications. These are often related to excessive volume, excessive pressure, and excessive FiO2 causing baro/volutrauma and/or lung injury. Ultimately, they will manifest as hypoxia and/or pneumothorax, pneumomediastinum, or subcutaneous emphysema. Adequate sedation, use of lowest effective tidal volume, and careful monitoring of pressures may help to prevent lung injury. Ventilator associated pneumonia develops in up to 28% of patients on MV; in-hospital mortality is approximately 50% with a similar mortality at 5 years after discharge. Prevention, recognition, and adequate treatment are obvious priorities.

INVASIVE MECHANICAL VENTILATION

A C U T E M A N A G E M E N T

The goal of mechanical ventilation is to optimize oxygenation and ventilation without causing harm.

Indications:

- To protect the airway (from obstruction, increased secretions, or loss of consciousness)
- Respiratory failure—increased work of breathing may worsen myocardial ischemia.
- Failed NIMV

Pearls of Mechanical Ventilation in Cardiac Care Unit (CCU)

- Provide sufficient oxygen to reverse hypoxic vasoconstriction, $\approx SaO_2$ 96%.
- Utilize the smallest tidal volume necessary to eliminate carbon dioxide
- Avoid patient-ventilator asynchrony with adequate sedation and analgesia (Fig. 31.1)
- Reduce work of breathing
- Recognize effects of positive-end expiratory pressure

Labs: Check a stat CMP, CBC, PT/PTT, and ABG with lactate

- Check portable CXR

Surgical: Tracheostomy can be considered after 7 days of mechanical ventilation and when extubation is not anticipated before 14 days.

CCU Tip: When positive-end expiratory pressure is applied in the presence of unilateral disease (i.e., pneumonia), it may worsen the V/Q mismatch, and thus worsen hypoxia and hypercarbia. Additionally, it can decrease preload and impair cardiac output thus causing hemodynamic instability.

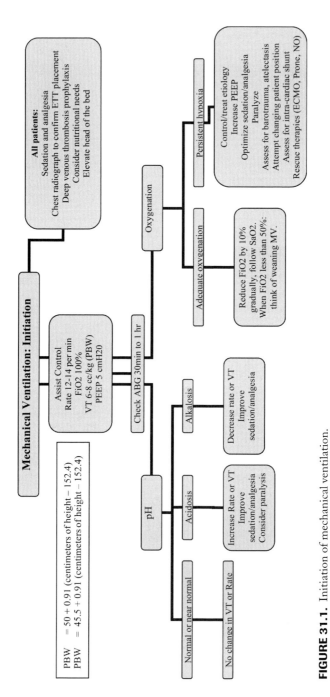

FIGURE 31.1. Initiation of mechanical ventilation.
PBW, Predicted Body Weight (Kgs); VT, tidal volume; ETT + Endotracheal tube; PEEP, Positive End Expiratory Pressure.

MECHANICAL VENTILATION TROUBLESHOOTING

- High peak pressure and no change in plateau pressure (or >10 mmH$_2$O difference) is often caused by increased resistance (ETT obstruction, bronchospasm, mucus plugging).
- High plateau pressures (>35 cmH$_2$O) are typically due to poor compliance. Frequent causes are high tidal volume, auto positive-end expiratory pressure, pneumothorax, large effusion, stiff lungs (ARDS, pneumonia, pulmonary fibrosis), or increased abdominal pressure (ascites).
- Persistent hypoxemia is most often due to extreme V/Q mismatch. Examples are PE, pneumonia, pulmonary edema, airway abstruction, or autoPEEP. Consider anatomical shunts (cardiac or pulmonary) when no pulmonary abnormality is present.
- AutoPEEP is classically seen in patients with asthma or chronic obstructive pulmonary disease, but also when a short expiratory time is used. It causes hyperinflation and air-trapping. This can be diagnosed by measuring the pressure at the end of an expiratory pause maneuver, or simply detach the ventilator from the ETT and assess the hemodynamic response. Treatment includes management of bronchospasm, reducing inspiratory time, increasing expiratory time, improving sedation, and/or paralysis (Figs. 31.2 and 31.3).

WEANING FROM MV

After resolving the need for MV, the patient should be assessed for weaning. If ready, a spontaneous breathing trial (SBT) should take place. The decision for extubation is made when clinical and safety endpoints (see the following) are achieved. Multiple parameters and measurements to predict successful weaning have been studied, most with variable performance in daily practice. A successful SBT is still the best assessment available to predict extubation. In cardiac patients, the increased work of breathing and increased venous return from a SBT may precipitate heart failure. The work of breathing imposed by the ETT can be enough to make the SBT fail. Some patients will do better with straight extubation. Intravenous afterload therapy may be considered transiently during extubation to prevent hypertensive flash pulmonary edema and re-intubation.

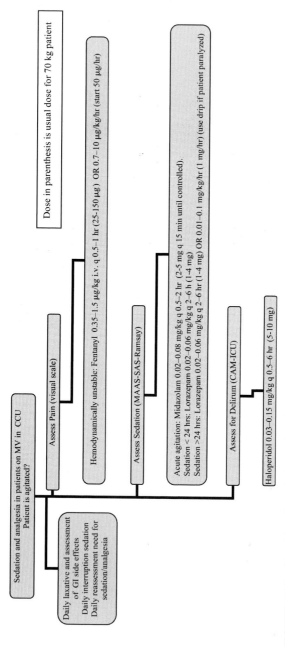

FIGURE 31.2. Algorithm for sedation and analgesia for mechanically ventilated patients in the Cardiac Care Unit.

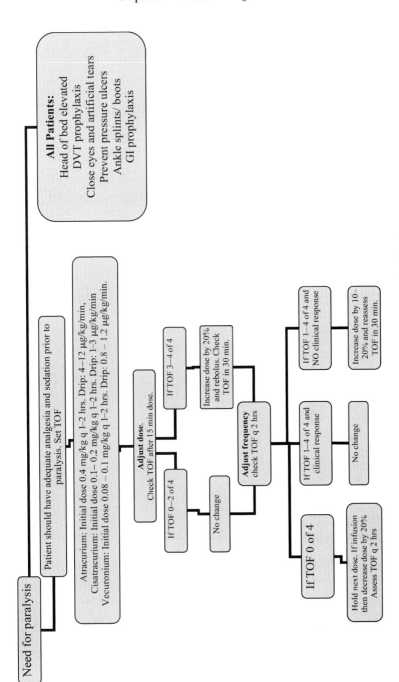

FIGURE 31.3. Algorithm for paralysis in the Cardiac Care Unit mechanically ventilated patients. TOF, Train of Four.

WEANING AND EXTUBATION

- Parameters for weaning: Resolve or optimize precipitating event. Patient aware and awake. Afebrile. Hemodynamic stability. FiO2 <50% (PaO2/FiO2 ratio >150), PEEP <5 mmH20, minute volume of <10 L/min.
- SBT trials: no sedation, or paralytic agent. ETT to T-piece or PS 7 mmH20/CPAP trial. 30 minute to 2 hour trial. Evaluate during and at the end of the trial.
- Failed SBT trial: The SBT is considered to have failed if the patient develops persistent hypoxemia, hypercarbia, acidosis, persistent tachypnea (RR >40 breaths/min) or hypotension. Other clues signaling imminent failure are hypertension, tachycardia, use of accessory muscles, diaphoresis and/or agitation. If a SBT is failed, then reinstitute full MV support for 24 hours before reattempting. If patient passes his SBT, then extubate if following criteria are met.
- Extubation criteria: Awake, FiO2 <50% with saturations >90%, RR <35, secretions being suctioned >2 hours and able to cough and has cuff leak when tested.
- After extubation: High-risk patients for re-intubation (i.e., hypercapnia, CHF, more than one failure of a weaning trial) may benefit from NIMV. Continue treatment of underlying condition and if possible aggressive control of afterload. Continue bronchodilator therapy if underlying lung disease.

INABILITY TO WEAN

If patient fails SBT trial, evaluate the cause: oxygenation, ventilation, or both.

Optimize the chances to wean by:

- Decreasing the work of breathing as much as possible (bronchodilation, decrease abdominal distension, consider drainage of pleural effusions, assess for myocardial ischemia, control fever, correct acid-base disorders, control pain, correct anemia).
- Optimizing nutrition.
- Assess for occult factors: hypothyroidism, hypophosphatemia, hypomagnesemia, diaphragmatic weakness/paralysis, muscle weakness and metabolic acidosis.

SEDATION IN THE CARDIAC PATIENT ON MV

Indication

- Decrease pain and anxiety, improve tolerance and comfort of MV, reducing the stress response and facilitating nursing care.

Contraindication

- Inability to protect airway and allergy.

Side Effects

- Hypotension frequently occurs in patients who have a decreased preload.
- Opioid mediated hypotension in euvolemic patients is a result of the combination of sympatholysis, vagally mediated bradycardia, and in the case of morphine, histamine release. Fentanyl and hydromorphone have the least hemodynamic effects.

TIP: Daily awakening of the patient, with reinitiating sedation at half the given dose reduces the time on MV (Fig. 31.2).

PARALYTIC AGENTS IN THE CARDIAC PATIENT

Indications

- Paralytic agents are used frequently as part of rapid sequence intubation. Other uses are to facilitate MV and to decrease oxygen consumption. They should also be used if optimal sedation/analgesia is unable to achieve the desired effects.

Contraindications

- Patient not sedated, allergy to paralytic agents, or a preexistent myopathy/neuropathy.

Side Effects

- Prolonged muscle weakness, muscle atrophy, venous thrombosis, pressure ulcers, corneal ulcers, and nerve compression. The cardiovascular side effects of paralytics include histamine release causing vasodilation and hypotension, vagal block causing tachycardia and ganglionic blockade causing hypotension. Use intermediate neuromuscular blockers (NMBs) with minimal cardiovascular effects.

RECOMMENDED READING

1. Nadar S, Prasad N, Taylor RS, et al. Positive pressure ventilation in the management of acute and chronic cardiac failure: a systematic review and meta-analysis. *Int J Cardiol.* 2005; 99:171–185

2. Pinsky MR. Cardiovascular issues in respiratory care. *Chest.* 2005; 128: 592S–597S.

3. Jacobi J, Fraser GL, Coursin DB, et al. Clinical practice guidelines for the sustained use of sedatives and analgesics in the critically ill adult. *Crit Care Med.* 2002; 30:119–141.

4. Murray MJ, Cowen J, DeBlock H, et al. Clinical practice guidelines for sustained neuromuscular blockade in the adult critically ill patient. *Crit Care Med.* 2002; 30:142–156.

CHAPTER 32

Sedation and Analgesia in the Coronary Intensive Care Unit

MICHAEL A. MILITELLO

Sedation is one of the most challenging issues encountered by critical care practitioners. There are multiple indications for sedation and the choice of sedative should be based on the needs and comorbidities of the individual patient. Some of the pitfalls of intensive care unit (ICU) sedation include failure to objectively assess the level of sedation, failure to individualize the approach to sedation, and failure to communicate sedation goals to other healthcare professionals. In this chapter, we will discuss general issues regarding sedation and analgesic use in the cardiac intensive care unit (CICU); in Chapter 31 we discuss sedation and paralytic use in intubated patients.

INDICATIONS FOR SEDATION

Sedation is essential because it provides patient comfort, prevent patients from harming themselves, and helps facilitate medical procedures. The choice of sedation technique depends on the clinical situation. A rudimentary approach in assessing an agitated patient is to think about the following four questions:

- Is the patient anxious?
- Is the patient in pain?
- Is the patient suffering from delirium?
- Is the patient sleep deprived?

Answering these four questions will help to direct both nonpharmacologic and pharmacologic approaches to caring for ICU patients. Other patient-specific considerations include mechanical ventilation, the need for procedures, and the use of intra-aortic balloon counterpulsation.

Treatment options for sedation should be directed toward patient-specific factors. Commonly used agents include benzodiazapines, narcotic analgesics, propofol, antipsychotic agents, and dexmedatomidine.

Sedative Agents

Benzodiazepines

Benzodiazepines are sedative-hypnotic agents that exert their anxiolytic and calming effects via $GABA_A$ receptor binding. This potentiates the effects of GABA and results in sedation, hypnosis, anesthesia, anticonvulsant effects, muscle relaxation, and respiratory depression. Drugs in this class are also useful in patients with a history of ethanol abuse as they can attenuate withdrawal symptoms and prevent delirium tremens. Benzodiazepines do not produce analgesia; however, they should be considered first-line therapy in patients experiencing agitation.

Drugs in the benzodiazepine class have very different pharmacokinetic profiles; awareness of these differences will assure safer and more effective sedation. The majority of ICUs commonly use lorazepam or midazolam. Table 32.1 describes the pharmacokinetic and pharmacodynamic data for specific benzodiazepines. Although both agents are used for short- and long-term sedation, there are important differences that should be emphasized. Lorazepam is the preferred drug for long-term ICU sedation. The advantages of lorazepam include its lack of active metabolites and intermediate duration of action. A disadvantage of lorazepam is a slower onset of action, which may not be ideal when a patient is acutely agitated. In addition, the propylene glycol diluent used for intravenous lorazepam may accumulate in the bloodstream leading to acute tubular necrosis and hyperosmotic metabolic acidosis. Propylene glycol toxicity typically occurs in patients receiving high doses of lorazepam for prolonged periods of time. In contrast, midazolam is a rapidly acting benzodiazepine with a short duration of action, ideal for acutely agitated patients. However, accumulation of midazolam and its active metabolites may lead to prolonged sedation. Several factors predispose patients to prolonged sedation with midazolam including renal failure, heart failure, obesity, and the use of medications that inhibit the cytochrome P 450 isoenzyme 3A4. Because of these limitations, midazolam is not the preferred benzodiazepine for long-term (>48 hours) sedation in critically ill patients.

Analgesic Agents

Opiates

Opiates are adjunctive therapy in acutely agitated patients when a pain syndrome is known or suspected. Many times these agents are incorrectly

Table 32.1	Pharmacology of benzodiazepines.					
Drug	Onset after IV Dose	Half-Life*	Metabolism	Intermittent Dose	Infusion Dose Range
Benzodiazepines					
Diazepam	2–5 min	20–120 h	Hepatic: active and inactive compounds	2–5 mg q 4–6 h	no
Lorazepam	5–20 min	12–15 h	Hepatic: inactive compounds	1–4 mg q 2–6 h	1–10 mg/h
Midazolam	1–5 min	2–6 h	Hepatic: active and inactive compounds	0.5–5 mg q 0.5–2 h	1–15 mg/h

* Parent compound

used as an alternative to sedatives. Although their use should be restricted to patients requiring pain control, opiates are often used in combination with sedatives, because it is frequently difficult to discern whether an agitated, noncommunicative patient is also experiencing pain. Basic pharmacologic and pharmacokinetic effects of commonly used opiates are reviewed in Table 32.2.

The opiate most commonly used for the treatment of pain in cardio-vascular patients is morphine sulfate. Morphine sulfate produces analge-sia and anxiolytic effects as well as arterial and venous vasodilatation, features that make it particularly well suited for the management of flash pulmonary edema. Common morphine side effects include nausea and vomiting. Hypotension can occur and is thought to be related to hista-mine release. As a result, morphine should be used cautiously in patients presenting with right-ventricular (RV) infarctions or in patients with suspected low intravascular volume. Other opiates such as fentanyl are more potent than morphine and cause less histamine release and there-fore less frequent hypotension. Adverse events associated with all opiates include constipation, respiratory depression, and blurred vision. Addi-tionally, morphine may cause miosis. Care should be taken to assure that all patients receiving opiates have an appropriate bowel regimen to pre-vent constipation.

Propofol

Propofol is a general anesthetic agent with a poorly understood mecha-nism of action. It has both sedative and hypnotic properties but does not produce analgesia. Propofol has a rapid onset of action and short dura-tion of effect. It is an ideal agent in patients who require frequent neuro-logical assessment and as bridge to extubation. IV-loading doses of propofol may cause significant hypotension and myocardial depression and should be avoided in hemodynamically unstable patients or in con-gestive heart failure (CHF). Typical infusion doses of propofol range from 5 to 50 µg/kg/min. Propofol is insoluble in aqueous vehicles and is available as a lipid emulsion with a caloric density of 1.1 kcal/mL. This should be considered when calculating caloric intake. Also, because propofol is available as a lipid emulsion, the manufacturer recommends administration through a dedicated intravenous line with intravenous tubing replaced every 12 hours. High-dose (>80 µg/kg/min) and/or long-term infusions have lead to hypertriglyceridemia and pancreatitis. Therefore, serum triglyceride levels should be obtained after 2 days of therapy. Other adverse effects are hypotension, bradycardia, respiratory depression, and myocardial depression. In our institution, propofol is

Table 32.2	Pharmacology and pharmacokinetics of selected opiates.				
Drug	Dosing	Onset (min)	Duration (h)	Half-life (h)	Elimination
Fentanyl	50–400 μg/h	1–5	0.5–1	~3	hepatic
Morphine	1–10 mg/h or 2–4 mg every 2–4 h as needed	10–20	2–4	3–4	hepatic/renal
Hydromorphone*	0.5–2 mg every 4–6 h as needed	15	4–5	2–3	hepatic

*Multiple errors in dosing have occurred and initiating at lowest dose is recommended.

rarely used in the CICU. In general, it should be used cautiously in patients with low ejection fraction, moderate to severe aortic stenosis, CHF, and in the setting of myocardial infarction (MI).

Antipsychotic Agents

Agents in this class of medications should be reserved for patients experiencing delirium. By blocking dopamine neurotransmission in the central nervous system, these agents may stabilize cerebral function. The most commonly used antipsychotic is haloperidol, which produces mild to moderate sedation. However, haloperidol may also produce extrapyramidal effects, neuroleptic malignant syndrome, acute dystonic reaction, and akathisia and may reduce seizure thresholds and induce QTc interval prolongation. Most case reports of significant electrocardiographic changes occur at dose greater than 50 mg daily in patients at risk of arrhythmias. Therefore, it should be used at low doses and cautiously in patients with underlying heart disease. It should also be avoided in patients on medications known to prolong the QTc interval such as Class Ia and III antiarrhythmic medications.

CLINICAL PRESENTATION TIPS

- Acute agitation can be intervened very effectively with midazolam due to its short onset of action.
- Pain in cardiac patients should be managed carefully. Hypotension may be induced and the etiology of the pain should be identified prior to utilizing opiate analgesia.
- Delirium can be treated with haloperidol, however, avoid in patients with prolonged QTc intervals and other QT prolonging medications such as selected antiarrhythmics.
- Respiratory failure should be considered in opiate overdose. If intubation is required propofol is generally avoided due to its hypotensive, bradycardiac, and myocardial depressant effects.
- Renal failure may be due to acute tubular necrosis induced by the diluent utilized in lorazepam—propylene glycol—and cause a metabolic acidosis.

RECOMMENDED READING

1. Jacobi J, et al. Clinical practice guidelines for the sustained use of sedatives and analgesics in the critically ill adult. [see comment] [erratum appears in *Crit Care Med* 2002 Mar;30(3):726]. *Crit Care Med.* 2002; 30(1):119–141.

2. Nasraway SA, Jr., et al. Sedation, analgesia, and neuromuscular blockade of the critically ill adult: revised clinical practice guidelines for 2002. *Crit Care Med.* 2002; 30(1):117–118.
3. Lawrence KR, NS. Conduction disturbances associated with administration of butyrophenone antipsychotics in the critically ill: a review of the literature. *Pharmacotherapy.* 1997; 17(3):531–537.

CHAPTER 33

Nutrition in the Coronary Care Unit

EMILY G. CHHATRIWALLA

Malnutrition in hospitalized patients is common, affecting 30% to 50% of patients, and is particularly detrimental in the intensive care unit (ICU) where it increases length of mechanical ventilation (MV), duration of ICU care, and overall mortality. Nutrition in the coronary care unit (CCU) most often involves the provision of enteral nutrition (EN) support because of the frequent need for MV. The initiation and management of EN as well as the indications for parenteral nutrition will be discussed here.

NUTRITION ASSESSMENT

Nutrition assessment is a comprehensive evaluation of a patient's nutritional status and should be performed when initiating nutrition support. A consult to nutrition therapy ensures that patients will receive appropriate evaluation of their nutritional needs and on-going monitoring of nutritional therapy. Visceral proteins such as albumin and prealbumin are negative acute phase reactants and therefore are not reliable indicator of nutritional status in the ICU patient population.

A variety of methods are used to estimate calorie and protein requirements. The easiest and most useful method uses kilograms of dry body weight to calculate calorie and protein needs. Critically ill patients usually require 20 to 30 kcals/kg/day and 1.5 to 2.0 grams of protein/kg/day. Overfeeding is a common complication of nutritional support and can lead to complications such as hyperglycemia, electrolyte abnormalities, hypercapnia, and infection. The goal of enteral feeding in the ICU is not to meet energy expenditure but rather to provide sufficient protein for

ACUTE MANAGEMENT

Estimated Energy Requirements in Patients

BMI 25–29	20–25 Kcal/kg dry weight
BMI 30–34.9	15–20 Kcal/kg dry weight
BMI ≥35	10–15 Kcal/kg dry weight

Management:

- **Tools:** Small bore feeding tube (i.e., Corpak) or large bore salem sump (i.e., NG tube)
- **Labs:** CMP, PT, INR, PTT, weight; also monitor gastric residuals and abdominal exam
- Sample enteral nutrition order:
  - Replete with fiber via corpak @ 30 mL/hr × 4 h
  - Advance by 20 mL/hr every 4 h to goal of 80 mL/h, as tolerated
  - HOB @ 30 degrees during tube feeding
  - check gastric residuals every 4 h. If >200 mL, hold feeding and notify doctor
  - 30 mL of water every 8 h via corpak

Surgical: Consider peg tube if prolonged nutrition is necessary.

CCU Tip: Early enteral nutrition is recommended if the patient cannot tolerate by mouth intake.

Adapted with permission from Parekh NR, DeChicco RS, eds. *Nutrition Support Handbook.* Cleveland, Ohio: Cleveland Clinic; 2004.

increased amino acid turnover while avoiding complications from excess total calories—so called "permissive underfeeding."

ENTERAL NUTRITION

EN refers to the provision of a patient's daily nutrition requirements via a formula infused through a feeding tube into the gastrointestinal (GI) tract. The first step in providing EN is to obtain enteral access.

Patients without underlying gastric dysmotility will likely tolerate gastric feeding well. Access to the stomach is also easier to obtain and nasogastric tubes are easier to replace should a tube become displaced. Consideration should be given to nasoenteric feeding in cases of delayed gastric emptying—i.e., pre-existing gastroparesis or persistently high gastric residuals (>200 mL), or high risk for aspiration, i.e., prolonged prone positioning. Patients who develop acute pancreatitis can be safely fed into the GI tract via a nasojejunal tube whose tip lies beyond the ligament of Treitz. Because of the difficulty in placing nasoenteric feeding tubes and the high risk for tube displacement, nasal bridles are a useful modality that can increase nutrition delivery and potentially improve patient care.

Once enteral access has been obtained and verified by x-ray, consideration should be given to the most appropriate enteral formula. In general, patients with a functional GI tract should be fed a standard 1 cal/mL polymeric formula. A wide variety of disease-specific formulas are available but are usually not indicated for the cardiac patient. However, in cases of fluid restriction, consideration should be given to a concentrated 1.5 or 2 cal/mL formula.

Once the formula has been selected, the starting and goal rate should be calculated. For most patients, it is safe to start at a rate between 30 to 50 mL/hr and advance as tolerated to goal, keeping in mind that most patients will not and likely do not need to meet goal within the first few days of illness.

Table 33.1	Indications for parenteral nutrition.

- GI Tract is inaccessible or unsafe for enteral nutrition
- Nonfunctional GI tract
  - Short bowel syndrome
  - Severe malabsorption
  - Obstruction or ileus
  - Intractable vomiting or diarrhea
  - Persistent, uncontrolled GI bleed
  - Radiation enteritis
  - Bowel ischemia
  - High-output fistula
  - Severe pancreatitis and unable to obtain/maintain enteral access
  - Severe colitis
  - Graft-versus-host disease of the gut

GI, gastrointestinal

SURGICAL EVALUATION

Long-term nutrition support is rare in the ICU population; however, in cases of prolonged MV requiring tracheotomy, concurrent long-term enteral access should be considered. Long-term enteral access improves patient comfort and can be achieved by placing a gastrostomy or jejunostomy tube.

CLINICAL PRESENTATION TIPS

- Aspiration: usually due to improper positioning (i.e., head of bed <30°). Also consider high gastric residuals or altered gag reflex.
- Diarrhea: infectious process such as C. diff or bacterial overgrowth, also consider malabsorption, too rapid infusion, bacterial contamination of formula, liquid medication containing sorbitol.
- Constipation: lack of fiber, inadequate fluid intake, fecal impaction, narcotics, ileus/altered mobility.
- Bloating/Cramping: may be secondary to rapid infusion rate, formula intolerance, bowel obstruction, ileus, or gastroparesis.
- Dehydration: osmotic diarrhea, excessive protein or electrolytes, or inadequate fluid intake.

COMPLICATIONS

- **High gastric residuals** result from delayed gastric emptying, prone positioning abdominal surgery, opiates, or anticholinergics and can result in emesis and/or aspiration. This should be addressed with a decreased rate of EN and checking the placement of the feeding tube by radiography and elevating the head of bed.
- **Infectious diarrhea** may occur with prolonged antibiotic use and needs to be evaluated with stool cultures and treatment of the underlying pathogen.
- **Refeeding syndrome** may occur in a chronically malnourished patient receiving calories via EN, PN, or IV fluids too rapidly. Electrolytes should be monitored regularly in patients on EN and replenished as necessary.

- **Volume overload** is particularly concerning in the CCU population especially in patients with heart failure. A concentrated, volume-restricted formula can prevent this problem.
- **Malabsorption** can occur with pancreatitis and should be addressed with pancreatic enzymes. If steatorrhea occurs, a lower fat formula may be utilized or a formula high in medium chain triglycerides.
- **Insulin resistance** is a common complication of critical illness that can be exacerbated by nutritional support. Patients receiving nutrition support in the CCU should be closely monitored for hyperglycemia and controlled with the use of subcutaneous sliding scale insulin; an insulin drip should be considered in cases of particularly erratic blood glucose levels.

RECOMMENDED READING

1. Shopbell J, Hopkins B, Shronts E. Nutrition screening and assessment. In: Gottschlich MM, ed. *The Science and Practice of Nutrition Support.* A Case-Based Core Curriculum. Dubuque: Kendall/Hunt Publishing Company; 2001:107–140.
2. Artinian V, DiGiovine B. The effects of early enteral feeding on the clinical outcomes of critically ill patients. *Chest.* 2003; 124:175S.
3. McClave SA, Greene LM, Snider HL, et al. Comparison of the safety of early enteral vs parenteral nutrition in mild acute pancreatitis. *JPEN.* 1997; 21:14–20.
4. Van den Berghe G, Wouters P, Weekers F, et al. Intensive insulin therapy in the surgical intensive care unit. *N Engl J Med.* 2001; 345:1359.

CHAPTER 34

Ethics in the Coronary Care Unit

ADNAN K. CHHATRIWALLA

Patients admitted to the Coronary Care Unit (CCU) are usually acutely ill and have high rates of morbidity and mortality. Patients with myocardial infarction, aortic dissection, or cardiogenic shock admitted to the CCU require immediate medical management, and the urgent admission or transfer of patients to the CCU often leads to gaps in communication between patient-care teams, patients, and their families. Even in situations in which medical care and medical or surgical procedures may be deemed "urgent" or "emergent," it is important that every effort be made to communicate effectively with patients and their families and to obtain informed consent for medical care and medical or surgical procedures. In many cases, care is further complicated when patients are unable to provide consent themselves. In these cases, the patient-care team must turn to patient surrogates to aid in decision making. Decisions regarding the continuation or withdrawal of aggressive medical care are perhaps the most difficult for patients and their loved ones as well as for physicians. Although numerous consultants and care-givers may influence the decisions made for any given patient, it is the job of the CCU team to tactfully present all relevant information to patients and their families, facilitate discussion of difficult issues and provide emotional support to patients and their families as needed.

COMMUNICATION

The ability of CCU physicians to communicate with patients and their families is essential to patient satisfaction. When patients are urgently transferred to the CCU, they usually arrive to the hospital well before their family members, who are almost invariably uninformed and worried. Although medical stabilization of patients must be the primary priority of CCU physicians, proper communication with patients' families is an essential step once the patient has been stabilized. Often times the best way for physicians to communicate with patients' families is through "family meetings." These can be impromptu or scheduled as the patient's hospital course dictates. If a patient is able to participate in such a meeting, then it may be held at the patient's bedside; if a patient is unable to participate, then it is often easier to hold a meeting in an available conference room. The advantages of formal family meetings include the ability of the patient-care team to more effectively convey information to several family members at once. During a family meeting, it is beneficial for the patient-care team to discuss the patient's clinical status and prognosis as well as to provide information regarding the current management plan and potential future plans. When discussing medical issues with patients and family members who are not in the medical field, it may be helpful to state the relevant issues more than once, and in different language, to increase understanding. In addition to the physician team, the presence of nursing staff involved in a patient's care and ancillary staff, e.g., a social worker, may be beneficial during such meetings.

INFORMED CONSENT

While it is common for physicians to document patients' "informed consent" before undertaking medical procedures and administration of blood products, the concept of informed consent is not limited to these specific situations. Informed consent refers to the notion that patients (and their families) should be active participants in their health care, and fully informed of their medical situation, prognosis, and potential risks and benefits of all therapeutic options prior to medical decision making. Therefore, it is important for physicians in the CCU to discuss not only current management with patients and their families, but also alternatives to current management. Patients and their families must be allowed to express their wishes as to the direction of their health care, and this may apply to the level of aggressiveness of their overall care as well as consent or refusal of specific procedures or therapies. While it is important to document a patient's informed consent in the hospital chart (all important issues pertaining to patient care should be documented), the concept of informed consent is a broad one that should guide all patient-management decisions.

DECISION MAKING

Strictly speaking, under the concept of informed consent, caregivers should provide information and therapeutic options to patients who would utilize the information to make their own decisions regarding their medical care. Patients themselves should make decisions regarding their medical care if they are able to do so, and, on occasion, the CCU team may need to assess a patient's competency. There is no single test which establishes a patient's competency to make medical decisions; rather, the physician team must make an assessment of patients' ability to think rationally, their understanding of their medical condition, and their understanding of treatment options as well as the consequences of each. Expert consultation from a psychiatric team may be obtained if there is difficulty in assessing a patient's competency.

In cases in which a patient is unable to make medical decisions, either due to unresponsiveness or incompetence, authority to make medical decisions becomes a legal issue that may be handled differently in different states or countries. Health-care providers should follow advance directives, if available. These are directions pertaining to medical care, issued by patients prior to their episode of unresponsiveness or incompetence. In most cases, however, even previously issued advance directives are somewhat vague and are not helpful in making day-to-day decisions in the CCU. In cases in which advance directives are unavailable or not helpful, medical decisions must be made by a patient proxy or patient surrogate, the legal definition of which may differ depending on the state or country. A patient proxy is a person (who may not be a family member) legally appointed by a patient to make medical decisions in situations in which the patient cannot. If a patient proxy has not previously been appointed, a patient surrogate is able to make medical decisions on a patient's behalf. In the United States, an adult patient's next of kin (often a spouse) would serve as the patient's surrogate if he or she is able to. It is important to provide surrogate decision makers with the information they need to make informed decisions on behalf of patients, as well as the emotional support they need to make such decisions, which are often difficult as they deal with a family member or friend's illness.

Rarely, there may exist conflict between the CCU team and patients or their families with regard to the best management plan for a patient. These situations must be dealt with very carefully, as it is important for everyone involved to not allow personal emotions to interfere with patient care. Conflict may also be seen between family members with differing opinions as to the best direction of patient care. Often times, conflict situations arise in situations involving end-of-life decisions. It is important to realize that family members may not have a full understanding of a patient's clinical course at the end of life. Furthermore, family members who have previously been told to remain hopeful may have difficulty adjusting when informed that a patient's condition is now terminal. Often times in such situations, conflicts can be more easily resolved after patients and their families have had time to reflect on new circumstances. One of the more difficult scenarios involves cases in which a patient surrogate feels unable to make medical decisions or declines to make decisions by removing him- or herself from the patient-care environment, often staying unavailable for contact by the patient-care team. In extreme cases, it may be necessary to have a court-appointed patient guardian make decisions in lieu of a surrogate who is unable or unwilling to make decisions on a patient's behalf. With any conflict scenario, it is important for the patient-care team to remain unemotional and unbiased when offering information and recommendations. At many institutions, assistance from an ethics or social work team may facilitate discussion with family members in conflict.

END OF LIFE CARE

End-of-life care decisions are extremely difficult for patients and their families as well as patient-care teams. As with other medical decisions, the presence of advance directives may be useful in assessing a patient's prior wishes if he or she is unable to communicate with the patient-care team. The decision to withhold or withdraw life-sustaining therapy must be carefully considered in scenarios in which patients do not improve despite aggressive measures in the CCU. Such decisions may be based on an assessment that the potential risks of aggressive therapy outweigh the potential benefits. Alternatively, such decisions may be based on a patient's own wishes regarding aggressive therapy regardless of potential risks or benefits. A distinction must be made between the provision of life-sustaining therapies and the provision of futile care, defined as measures that are unlikely to provide benefit. Many patients and family members may struggle with issues of morality when dealing with end-of-life discussions and may wish to speak with a religious cleric, who is available on call at many hospitals.

Physician-assisted suicide is a controversial topic in the United States and remains illegal in most states, with the exclusion of Oregon. A chief concern with legalization of physician-assisted suicide is that such an option might be seen as an alternative for patients in poor, underserved (and uninsured) populations who wish to not place additional burdens on their families. A second concern involves the potential for caregivers to choose physician-assisted suicide as an alternative to medical care for patients who are unable to make decisions for themselves, and to thereby eliminate patients who place a higher-than-average burden on the medical system. Despite these concerns, physician assisted suicide is legal in some other countries, most notably the Netherlands. Should a patient request assistance in suicide from the CCU team, the most appropriate response should be to investigate and address potential reasons for the patient request, including inadequate pain management, depression, or delirium.

Depending on the patient's underlying state, the withholding or withdrawal of therapies such as mechanical ventilation, vasopressor support, or pacemaker may result in a patient's demise in relatively short fashion. If a decision to withhold therapy is agreed upon, patient comfort should be considered in the likely event that the patient expires quickly. This may include management of pain (which may be related to the underlying disease process as well as to therapeutic interventions) as well as treatment of anxiety and dyspnea. Pain-rating scales may be of benefit in allowing patients to more clearly describe the extent of any discomfort that they feel. In unresponsive patients, the CCU team may need to rely on indirect indicators of pain such as agitation, increased pulse, or increased blood pressure when assessing patient comfort. Family members who are present may also be able to assist the CCU care team in assessing patient comfort. The administration of morphine via IV push or continuous IV infusion is often beneficial in pain management. Dyspnea may or may not be related to underlying lung pathology at the end of life, and may respond well to morphine in addition to standard respiratory therapy with bronchodilator agents. Anticholinergic agents may be utilized to decrease oral secretions if this is felt to contribute to a patient's dyspnea. Benzodiazepine administration may alleviate patient anxiety, if present, and anti-emetics may be utilized for symptoms of nausea. As important as patient comfort is at the end of life, it is equally important to address the concerns of family and friends during end-of-life situations, and at our institution we are careful to avoid interruptions (e.g., monitor alarms, blood draws, too-frequent vital signs) in cases in which a patient's family wishes to spend time together in peace.

SUMMARY

While the urgent medical stabilization of patients is often of highest priority to patient-care teams in the CCU, ethical considerations should be stressed with equal importance. Despite the acuity of illness present in the CCU, care providers must respect patient autonomy and the concept of informed consent when making difficult management decisions. Good communication improves patient and family satisfaction with medical providers and can allow CCU patient-care teams to work more closely with patients and their families to make difficult medical decisions.

Case Presentation

CHAPTER 35

Ruptured Papillary Muscle with Acute Mitral Regurgitation

ESTHER S. H. KIM

BRIEF HISTORY

The patient is a 67-year-old active beef cattle farmer with no significant previous cardiac history. He is a nonsmoker, denies alcohol or illicit drug use, and is not on any medications. In June 2005, he presented to an outside institution with complaints of "bad taste in my mouth," anorexia, nausea, insomnia, increasing dyspnea, generalized fatigue, and a dry cough. He was diagnosed with atrial fibrillation with rapid ventricular rate, bilateral pneumonia, and elevated liver enzymes. An extensive work up included chest x-ray showing cardiomegaly and bilateral infiltrates, chest CT showing no pulmonary embolus but presence of patchy pneumonic infiltrates, right upper-quadrant ultrasound and colonoscopy, which were done for abdominal distention and read as normal. There was a question of a fungal pneumonia or pneumonitis given the patient's occupation as a farmer, and he was empirically treated with IV steroids. He was also started on antibiotics and diuretics, and he eventually improved to the point of discharge. Discharge medications included amoxicillin/clavulanate acid, doxycycline, bronchodilators, atenolol, digoxin, diltiazem, coumadin, and low-dose furosemide. An echocardiogram was ordered but results were not available at the time of discharge.

Ten days after discharge, the patient presents again to the outside emergency department. He complained of distended abdomen and increasing dyspnea. He was admitted with "recurrent pneumonia, dyspnea, dehydration."

EXAM

On exam, he was in distress with a temperature 38.2°C, blood pressure 120/70, pulse 80, respiratory rate 23 with O_2 sat of 95% on 100% nonrebreather mask (NRB). He was unable to speak in full sentences secondary to dyspnea, but no note of jugular venous distention was made. His cardiac exam showed regular rhythm, normal S1, S2, no murmurs, rubs, or gallops. His lung sounds were decreased bilaterally at the bases, and there were bilateral rales and extensive wheezing. His abdomen was noted to be distended but soft, and his extremities had no edema.

LABS

Labs showed creatinine 1.3, AST 39, ALT 76, lipase 320, amylase 78, WBC 15.6K with 82% neutrophils, INR 2.6. ECG showed atrial fibrillation with a rate of 88 and inferior t-wave inversions. Cardiac enzymes were negative.

MANAGEMENT

His presentation was thought to be consistent with a primary pulmonary process, and he was treated with intravenous antibiotics and steroids. Bronchoscopy was planned, but the patient was felt to be too unstable. Two days after admission, the patient worsened. His O_2 sat was 83% on 100% NRB, and he became hypotensive. He was intubated and a norepinephrine drip was started. His labs at this point were significant for AST 42, ALT 70, lipase 1252, amylase 340, creatinine 1.4, and WBC 20.8K with 95% neutrophils. A transesophageal echocardiogram was performed and showed an ejection fraction of 60% without regional wall-motion abnormalities, severe prolapse, and partial flail of the anterior leaflet of the mitral valve and rupture of the chordae tendinae. There was severe mitral regurgitation with demonstrable reversible flow within the pulmonary veins (Figs. 35.1 and 35.2).

The patient also had a cardiac catheterization that showed mild narrowing of the left main trunk, left anterior descending artery with severe stenosis of the mid and distal portions, a mid-sized first diagonal branch with a severe 90% proximal lesion, left circumflex artery with a proximal 75%, a distal 50% lesion, and a severe 70% lesion in a mid-sized second obtuse marginal branch. The right coronary artery also had a severe 75% mid-vessel lesion, and the right posterior descending artery also had a 50% mid-vessel lesion.

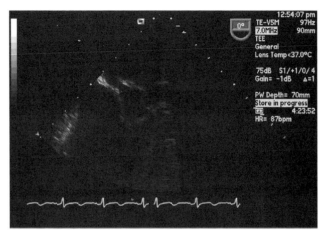

FIGURE 35.1. Transesophageal echocardiogram showing flail and prolapse of the medial portion of the anterior mitral valve secondary to chordal rupture.

The patient was diagnosed with cardiogenic shock, an intra-aortic balloon pump was inserted, and he was transferred to our cardiac care unit (CCU) for further medical management and evaluation for open heart surgery.

On arrival to the CCU, a pulmonary artery catheter was inserted and initial revealed the following: CI 3.17L/min/m^2, PA 72/49

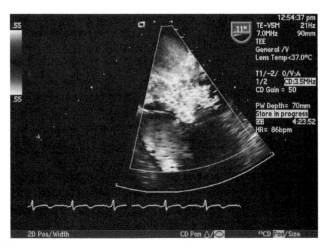

FIGURE 35.2. Transesophageal echocardiogram with color flow imaging showing posteriorly directed severe mitral regurgitation.

mmHg, CVP 20 mmHg, mean PCWP 30 mmHg, SvO_2 62%. Pulmonary artery tracing was significant for the presence of large V waves. The norepinephrine drip was weaned off within 1 hour of arrival, broad spectrum antibiotics were continued, and aggressive preload and afterload reduction was initiated with nitroglycerin and nitroprusside drips. A lasix drip was started and over the next 24 hours, the patient had a brisk diuresis of over three liters. Repeat hemodynamic numbers showed CI 3.4 L/min/m^2, PA 75/33 mmHg, CVP 22 mmHg, mean PCWP 20 mmHg, SvO_2 66%. The ventilator was able to be weaned to minimal settings. Bronchoscopy was performed and showed only normal respiratory flora and a few polymorphonuclear leukocytes. Serial blood cultures were negative, and after a total diuresis of 10 liters, the patient was considered to be stable for open heart surgery.

Visual inspection of the valve in the operating room demonstrated flail of the posterior half of the anterior leaflet with rupture of the posteromedial group of chordae to the anterior leaflet. A CE valve was inserted in the mitral position and a three-vessel CABG was performed (LIMA to LAD, SVG to lateral LCx, SVG-RCA). Pathology of the mitral valve showed myxomatous degeneration and no evidence of giant cells or granulomata. The papillary muscle had mild hypertrophy of the myocytes and no evidence of necrosis.

CCU TIPS

- Shortness of breath may be a manifestation of severe valvular dysfunction—a Swan-Ganz catheter can help define cardiogenic versus noncardiogenic pulmonary edema.
- Aggressive afterload reduction in acute mitral regurgitation is crucial. Norepinephrine can impair forward flow in the setting of mitral regurgitation.
- Rapid diagnosis and treatment of acute mitral regurgitation is critical.

EXPERT COMMENTARY

Although not a common manifestation of acute myocardial infarction (MI) in the reperfusion era, papillary muscle rupture is one of the most challenging for effective hemodynamic management as a bridge to surgery. In this case, the early missed diagnosis of the patient having a primary pulmonary problem rather than a catastrophic mitral-valve apparatus structural event could have easily led to the patient's rapid demise. As is often the case, the echo (in this patient a TEE) helped save the day by making the correct diagnosis.

CHAPTER 36

Fulminant EBV Myocarditis

THOMAS H. WANG

BRIEF HISTORY

A 26-year-old male with no significant past medical history presents with a 2-day history of shortness of breath. His past medical history is notable only for a history of borderline hypertension and recurrent sinusitis. He has no family history of premature coronary artery disease. He is on no medications, is a nonsmoker with rare alcohol intake, and denied illicit drug use. He runs one to two miles a day and recently returned from a cruise to Brazil 5 months prior to presentation.

EXAM

On physical exam, he is in acute distress with the following vital signs: temperature 39.5°C; heart rate 128 beats per minute; blood pressure 94/44; respiratory rate 35 breaths per minute; and O_2 saturation of 85%. His jugular venous pressure (JVP) is 10 cm of water, and there are rales diffusely bilaterally. His cardiac exam is notable for tachycardia, an S3, and a laterally displaced PMI but no murmurs or rubs are noted. His abdomen is benign. His extremities are cool have 1+ pitting edema.

LABS

An ABG shows a pH of 7.16 with pCO_2 of 60 and PO_2 of 27 and a lactic acid of 5.2. Stat labs reveal acute renal failure with a creatinine of 1.8. His WBC is 14.0 with a Hgb of 14.1 and Plts of 269. Cardiac enzymes are positive with a troponin I of 43.88. An ECG reveals ST elevations in leads V1 to V4 and also in I and AVL with some ST depression inferiorly. A TSH level is normal.

MANAGEMENT

The patient is emergently intubated and heparinized. A bedside echocardiogram reveals an EF of 15% with global hypokinesis and no significant valvular pathology. There is a small pericardial effusion but no clinical or echocardiographic evidence of tamponade. An emergent left-heart catheterization shows no angiographic evidence of atherosclerotic disease. The left ventricular function by ventriculography is 15% to 20%, and there is no significant mitral regurgitation. During the procedure, the patient has profound tachycardia with rates into the 140s and lopressor is administered. The patient's blood pressure drops precipitously, however, and an intra-aortic balloon pump is placed. Norepinephrine is started simultaneously.

A right-heart catheterization reveals severely elevated pulmonary pressure with PAP of 60/40 mmHg and a RAP of 30 mmHg. The PCWP is 30 to 35 mmHg. The cardiac output is 2.2 L/min with a cardiac index of 1.13 L/min. The patient is transported to the coronary care unit (CCU) in critical condition and subsequently supported with norepinephrine and milrinone, high-dose steroids and antibiotics.

While in the CCU, he becomes difficult to oxygenate and requires high levels of PEEP. His hemodynamics remain tenuous and a CXR reveals pneumomediastinum—bilateral chest tubes are then inserted. His renal failure worsens with a creatinine of 3.9, and he is transferred to our institution for consideration of a left-ventricular assist device and/or transplantation.

Upon arrival, his hemodynamics remain tenuous on milrinone and norepinephrine. However, these medications are able to be gradually weaned off in favor of afterload reduction with nitroprusside. His empiric steroids and antibiotics are continued. On this regimen, his oxygenation improves and his chest tubes are discontinued. Upon further review of his history, the patient had prodromal symptoms consisting of a sore throat, fatigue, and lymphadenopathy. An ebstein barr virus panel is sent and returns positive confirming the diagnosis of fulminant Epstein-Barr virus (EBV) myocarditis. The patient continues to improve on nitroprusside and is able to have his IABP discontinued on day 2 and is then extubated. A repeat echocardiogram on day 3 reveals normal left-ventricular function and no evidence of valvular disease. He is transitioned to oral ace inhibitors and beta blockers and does well after being transferred to a telemetry floor. He is subsequently discharged home.

He is later seen in follow up and is noted to have normal left-ventricular function with excellent recovery.

CCU TIPS

- Beware of beta-blockers in a compensatory tachycardia as they may precipitate cardiogenic shock!
- Myocarditis should be considered in the differential diagnosis of ST-segment elevations on ECG.
- Maximal medical support with an Swan-Ganz catheter, intra-aortic balloon pump, and vasoactive therapies are indicated in transient myocarditis.

EXPERT COMMENTARY

It is important to never forget that many things can masquerade as an myocardial infarcion (MI)—in this case myocarditis. Another noteworthy point is that we often cannot establish the root cause of a fulminant myocarditis—in this particular case EBV was the culprit and is known to have the capacity to induce a life-threatening, profound myocardial insult.

CHAPTER 37

Giant Cell Myocarditis in a Bone Marrow Transplant Recipient

GREGORY G. BASHIAN

BRIEF HISTORY

A 24 year-old male presented with low-grade fevers, jaw discomfort, and chest pain. His past medical history was notable for acute myeloid leukemia diagnosed 3 years prior to admission for which he received idarubicin and cytarabine chemotherapy. His leukemia relapsed requiring allogenic, matched, unrelated bone marrow transplantation 1 year prior to admission. His post-transplant course was notable for the development of graft-versus-host disease (for which he was treated with corticosteroids), steroid-induced diabetes mellitus, multiple deep venous thromboses, several bouts of acute renal failure, pancytopenia, and numerous infections.

His medical regimen consisted of prophylactic acyclovir, itraconazole, ciprofloxacin, and trimethoprim/sulfamethoxazole, in addition to his prednisone. Of note, he had self-discontinued his tacrolimus, and tapered his prednisone in the days prior to presentation.

LABS

Laboratories on admission were notable for chronic renal insufficiency (Cr = 1.7 mg/dL), anemia (Hgb = 9.5 g/dL), leukopenia (WBC = 2.9 K/μL), thrombocytopenia (PLT = 36 K/μL), and elevated cardiac biomarkers (Troponin-T = 1.64 ng/mL, CK = 92 U/L, MB = 18.1 ng/mL). Chest radiograph was normal. His admission electrocardiogram (ECG) demonstrated sinus tachycardia at 114 bpm; 1 to 2 mm ST-segment elevation with PR-segment depression in the inferior, lateral, and apical leads; and PR-elevation in lead aVR (Fig. 37.1). Echocardiography initially

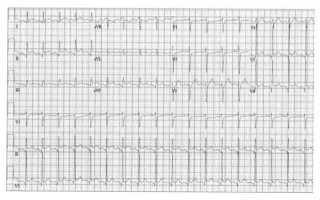

FIGURE 37.1. Admission electrocardiogram. Sinus tachycardia is seen with 1 to 2 mm ST-segment elevation and PR-segment depression in the inferior, lateral, and apical leads. There is also PR-segment elevation in lead aVR. This ECG is consistent with acute pericarditis.

demonstrated a low-normal left-ventricular systolic function with an ejection fraction of 50%, and a small to moderate circumferential pericardial effusion.

MANAGEMENT

The diagnosis of myopericarditis was made, the patient was continued on his corticosteroid regimen, and nonsteroidal anti-inflammatory drugs (NSAIDs) were added. He was also treated with intravenous hydration and broad-spectrum antibiotic, antifungal, and antiviral medications due to his fever and immunocompromised state.

On the 8th hospital day, the patient's condition worsened.

EXAM

Febrile to 38.4°C, tachycardic to 140 bpm with a regular rhythm, blood pressure (BP) 105/63. He is a lethargic, ill-appearing young male; there is obvious jugular venous distention (JVD); lungs with scattered rhonchi; a nondisplaced point of maximum impulse; an S3 without murmurs or rub; and cool extremities with bilateral lower-extremity pitting edema.

Electrocardiography demonstrated sinus tachycardia; diffuse ST-segment elevation greater than 5 mm in the anterior precordial leads; mild PR-depression; and PR-elevation in lead aVR (Fig. 37.2). Cardiac

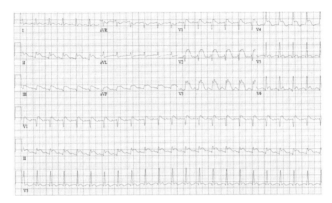

FIGURE 37.2. Hospital day #8 electrocardiogram. Sinus tachycardia is again seen, now to a rate of 140 bpm. There are also more profound ST-segment elevations in the inferior and now anterior leads.

biomarkers were further elevated (Troponin-T = 21.58 ng/mL, CK = 354 U/L, MB = 104.9 ng/mL). Echocardiography was notable for normal right-ventricular (RV) and left-ventricular (LV) size, severe RV and LV dysfunction with an LV ejection fraction of 10%, and a moderate pericardial effusion without evidence of tamponade (Fig. 37.3). Coronary angiography revealed normal coronary arteries.

The patient's intensive care unit (ICU) course was remarkable for the development of atrial fibrillation, as well as runs of nonsustained ventricular tachycardia. His renal failure worsened to a peak Cr of 3.2 with oliguria, and he became more hypoxic and lethargic. Pulmonary arterial (PA) catheterization was performed revealing the following pressures: PA = 21/16 and pulmonary capillary wedge pressure (PCWP) = 16 mmHg, with a HR = 101 bpm, and BP = 106/52 (MAP = 72 mmHg). Mixed venous oxygen saturation was 33%, giving a cardiac index of 1.73 L/min*m^2. He was treated with high doses of sodium nitroprusside after which his cardiac index improved to 2.81 L/min*m^2.

The patient was believed to have fulminant myopericarditis, and giant cell myocarditis was suspected due to the rapid decline in LV function and runs of ventricular tachycardia. Empiric high-dose corticosteroid therapy was initiated (methylprednisolone 1 gm IV daily for 3 days), and RV biopsy was obtained. The RV biopsy procedure induced sustained ventricular tachycardia requiring DC cardioversion, and was thus aborted after only one specimen was available for pathologic exam-

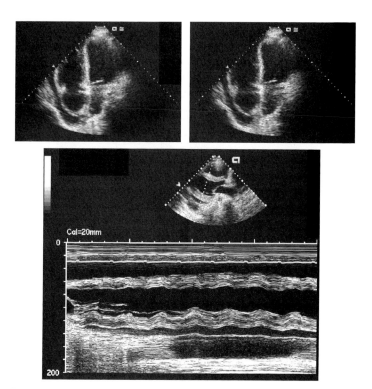

FIGURE 37.3. Hospital day #8 echocardiogram. Seen on the first row is the apical four chamber view at end-diastole and end-systole, respectively. Note the minimal contraction of the ventricles and the pericardial effusion. Depicted on the second row is an M-mode image of the horizontal short axis view demonstrating minimal excursion of the septum and posterior wall, as well as a pericardial effusion.

ination. Toluidine blue staining revealed a prominent inflammatory infiltrate, macrophages with vacuoles, diffuse necrosis, and giant cells (without evidence of caseating material), consistent with the diagnosis of giant cell myocarditis (Fig. 37.4).

Over the week following the high-dose corticosteroid and nitroprusside treatment, the patient's mental status, urine output, creatinine, hemodynamics, and ECG dramatically improved. LV function improved with an LV ejection fraction of 45% on subsequent echocardiography. The patient was ultimately discharged home.

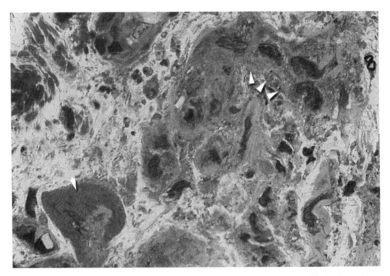

FIGURE 37.4. Toluidine blue staining of myocardial biopsy. Toluidine blue staining of the myocardial biopsy specimen demonstrates cardiac myocytes (arrow), as well as multinucleated giant cells (arrowheads) without evidence of caseating material. This is consistent with the diagnosis of giant cell myocarditis.

CCU TIPS

- A low threshold for myocardial biopsy in patients with subacute myocarditis is of great importance.
- Giant cell myoarditis should be considered in patients with rapid decline in left-ventricular function and ventricular arrhythmias.
- Aggressive immunosuppression with steroids prior to diagnosis may be necessary in severely decompensated patients

EXPERT COMMENTARY

This is a fascinating, rare cause of fulminate myocarditis. A tip-off can be the propensity for ventricular tachycardia. Compared with so many causes of myocarditis in which the biopsy is unhelpful, here the segue to effective therapy is essential.

CHAPTER 38

Right Ventricular Infarction

JOHN M. GALLA

BRIEF HISTORY

A 44-year-old white female nurse with a history of hypertension and current tobacco smoking not on any medications was in her usual state of health until the evening prior to presentation when she developed nausea and lightheadedness. The patient ignored these symptoms and, after a night of uneventful sleep, went to work. She collapsed several hours later and was found to be in ventricular fibrillation. After successful defibrillation, intubation, and stabilization; electrocardiography demonstrated ST elevation inferiorly; thus the patient was transferred by helicopter to the cardiac catheterization laboratory.

EXAM

On presenting exam, the patient was intubated with a blood pressure of 130/100 and a heart rate of 92. The lungs were clear to auscultation. The heartbeat was regular without any murmurs, rubs, or gallops. There were normal first and second heart sounds. The abdomen was soft, nontender and nondistended with a well-healed Pfannenstiel incision. There was no peripheral edema, clubbing, or cyanosis, and distal pulses were normal.

LABS

The patient's studies included a normal chemistry with the exception of a potassium level of 3.0 mmol/L, white blood cell count 13,900 (per mm^3), hematocrit 35.1 (%), and platelets 296,000 (per mm^3). The pro-thrombin time was normal, and the activated partial thromboplastin

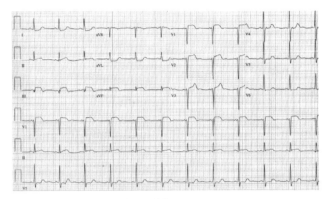

FIGURE 38.1. ECG with inferior ST elevations.

time was prolonged at 84.9 seconds. Cardiac enzymes showed an initial creatinine kinase of 2910, CK-MB 285, and Troponin T of 4.5. Portable chest radiography demonstrated a normal cardiac silhouette without pulmonary congestion. ECG revealed sinus rhythm with 3 to 4 mm ST-segment elevation in leads II, III, and aVF, normal axis and intervals (Fig. 38.1). A right-sided ECG was obtained which revealed ST-segment elevation in V4 indicative of a right-ventricular (RV) infarction (Fig. 38.2).

MANAGEMENT

The patient was brought directly from the helipad to the catheterization laboratory. Diagnostic cardiac catheterization revealed moderate coronary atherosclerosis in the left anterior descending and left circumflex arteries. The right coronary artery was totally occluded in the proximal third with the

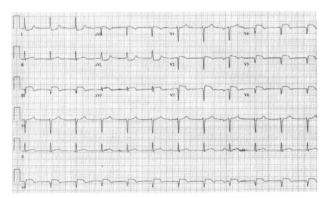

FIGURE 38.2. Right-sided ECG with ST elevation in V4.

angiographic appearance of fresh thrombus proximal to the RV marginal branch. After crossing the lesion with a guidewire and several passes with a thrombus extraction catheter, restoration of coronary circulation revealed a long proximal 70% stenosis, which was felt to be the culprit lesion. This was successfully stented with 3-drug-eluting stents and the patient was returned to the cardiac intensive care unit (ICU) in stable condition.

The patient was successfully extubated and begun on an oral regimen including beta blockade that afternoon in the cardiac intensive care unit (CICU). The patient subsequently became profoundly hypotensive and required re-intubation. Intravenous fluids were begun and a chest roentogram demonstrated clear lung fields without evidence of pulmonary vascular congestion. Bedside echocardiography demonstrated mild decrease in left-ventricular (LV) function, estimated ejection fraction 50%, moderate RV dysfunction with 3+ tricuspid regurgitation and an estimated RV systolic pressure of 33 mmHg.

A Swan-Ganz pulmonary artery catheter was placed via a left internal jugular approach. The pulmonary capillary wedge pressure was 16 mmHg and right-atrial pressure was 12 mmHg indicative of RV infarction physiology. Due to persistent hypotension, the patient was begun on an intravenous dobutamine. Following a protracted intensive-care course compliated by ventilator associated pneumonia and acute renal failure the patient was weaned off inotropic support, extubated, and made a full recovery.

CCU TIPS

- Right-sided ECGs should be obtained in inferior infarctions if there is concern for right-ventricular involvement.
- Swan-guided therapy may assist in right-ventricular infarct physiology due to the need for aggressive hydration and potential inotropic therapy.
- Patients with right-ventricular infarct may require long intensive-care-unit stay with supportive therapy, such as dobutamine.

EXPERT COMMENTARY

RV infarction is one of the most interesting and important acute myocardial infarction (MI) diagnoses, usually part of the "package" that needs to be considered with any inferior, posterior MI. The diagnosis of RV dysfunction is particularly vital, since it has such a dramatic effect on management compared with those infarcts with exclusive LV involvement.

CHAPTER **39**

Heparin-Induced Thrombocytopenia in a Cardiac Patient

DEBORAH KWON

BRIEF HISTORY

A 60-year-old female is postoperative day 8 from three-vessel CABG who presented to an outside hospital with hypotension, hypoxia, and right-sided hemiparesis. She had been a relatively healthy woman until November 2005 when she presented with progressive dyspnea on exertion without any chest pain. Her past medical history was remarkable for hypertension, obstructive sleep apnea, and hyperlipidemia. She was on atorvastatin 20 mg daily and hydrochlorothiazide 25 mg daily, and did not smoke, drink alcohol, or use illicit drugs. Her family history was notable only for hypertension and obesity. A routine stress test demonstrated ischemia in the anterior and lateral walls. She then underwent a left-heart catheterization that demonstrated severe 3-vessel disease. Based on this finding, she underwent coronary artery bypass grafting and did will postoperatively except for persistent hypoxia for which she was discharged on home oxygen.

At home, she had persistent shortness of breath with worsening diaphoresis and subsequently was found down in a confused state. Emergency medical service (EMS) was called, and she was rushed to an outside hospital.

EXAM

On physical exam, she was in acute distress with a temperature of 38.5°C, heart rate of 117, blood pressure of 72/54, respiratory rate of 32, and an oxygen saturation of 80% on 100% face mask. There was no jugular venous distention (JVD) with bilateral pulmonary rhochi.

No murmurs, rubs, or gallops were appreciated. Her abdomen was soft, mildly distended, with normoactive bowel sounds. Her neurologic exam was significant for decreased strength in her right upper and right lower extremity.

LABS

Her chemistries were normal except for potassium of 3.3 mg/dL, bicarbonate level of 29 mg/dL, BUN 32 mg/dL, Creatinine 1.6 mg/dL, and glucose 144 mg/dL. Her WBC was 20,200 (per mm^3), Hct 30.9 (%), and platelets 33,000 (per mm^3). Her INR and partial thromboplastin time were 1.2, and 29.6 seconds, respectively. Her CK was 76 U/L, CK-MB 4.9 ng/mL, and troponin-T 0.30 ng/mL. Her liver function tests were significant for AST 147 U/L, ALT 141 U/L, and Alkaline phosphatase 95 U/L. Her fibrinogen was 170 mg/d and D-dimer was >20,000 ng/mL.

A head CT demonstrated no signs of ischemia or bleeding. Patient continued to have signs of R-sided hemiplegia. A V/Q scan showed low-probability for pulmonary embolism (PE) but the patient continued to have profound hypoxia requiring 100% fractional inspired oxygen (FiO2). A TEE was performed revealing normal left-ventricular (LV) systolic function with right-ventricle (RV) dilatation. There was 2+ TR with a RV systolic pressure of 102 mmHg and a patent foramen ovale with right to left flow through the interatrial septum.

MANAGEMENT

Based on the patient's presentation, she was initially intubated, started on broad-spectrum antibiotics, and given a platelet transfusion for thrombocytopenia. Additionally, because a pulmonary embolism was suspected despite the low-probability V/Q scan, the patient was treated with empiric enoxaparin. She was then transferred to our institution.

Upon arrival, low-dose bivalirudin was started immediately due to the high suspicion of HITT as the patient's platelets were now 16,000. Heparin-induced platelet aggregation test and antiplatelet Factor 4 antibody ELISA was sent off immediately. A repeat head CT revealed a large acute left middle cerebral artery distribution infarct with mild localized mass effect. Upper- and lower-extremity Dopplers were then obtained that revealed acute deep-vein thrombosis of the right distal external iliac, right common femoral, right femoral, and right popliteal veins. Based on these findings, it was thought that the patient had developed DVTs secondary to HIT, which had embolized to her lungs and brain through her patent foramen ovale (PFO).

Her heparin-induced platelet aggregation test and antiplatelet Factor 4 antibody ELISA were indeed abnormal on the next day. Neurology was consulted to determine the risk for hemorrhagic conversion of the patient's stroke, which was deemed to be intermediate. Low-dose bivalirudin was continued to prevent further thrombosis while minimizing the risk of hemorrhagic conversion of her stroke. Additionally, a removable IVC filter was placed.

She gradually improved on this therapeutic regimen and was eventually successfully extubated. Her platelets slowly rose to over 50,000, and she recovered enough to be discharged home on oral anticoagulation.

CCU TIPS

- Maintain a high level of suspicion for HIT in patients post-CABG presenting with shortness of breath
- Severe thrombocytopenia and hypoxia should initiate a work up for HIT
- Anticoagulation with direct thrombin inhibitors in the setting of HIT and minimizing any possible heparin exposure can effectively minimize the thrombotic complications of HIT

EXPERT COMMENTARY

HIT certainly seems to be on the rise, perhaps in part to heightened awareness. Any patient on heparin who develops thrombocytopenia should at least be considered to have HIT until proven otherwise. The current case is particularly illustrative in the post-CABG setting with a presentation that could easily have been missed.

CHAPTER 40

Postpartum Cardiomyopathy

CARLOS A. HUBBARD

BRIEF HISTORY

A 21-year-old female develops acute respiratory distress with hypotension and tachycardia 1 day following an uncomplicated cesarean delivery after a normal full-term pregnancy. Her past medical history is unremarkable. She has no history of smoking, alcohol abuse, or drug abuse and is only taking prenatal vitamins. She requires emergent intubation and mechanical ventilation. A CT angiogram is negative for pulmonary embolus. An echocardiogram after intubation reveals severe left- and right-ventricular dysfunction with a left-ventricular (LV) ejection fraction of 10%. Also, severe LV dilatation with moderate mitral regurgitation is noted. She is started on vasopressors and ionotropes and develops elevated hepatic transaminases and oliguria with decreased creatinine clearance. Six days after delivery while on full respiratory support she suffers asystolic cardiac arrest and is resuscitated with epinephrine and atropine. She is then transferred to the Cleveland Clinic on norepinephrine and is receiving intravenous fluid boluses for hypotension.

EXAM

On admission to our institution, she is afebrile on full ventilatory support. A physical exam reveals a heart rate of 133 with a blood pressure of 118/62. She has prominent jugular venous distention (JVD), a regular heart rhythm with an S4 gallop, bilateral rales, scant bowel sounds and mild lower-extremity edema.

MANAGEMENT

A pulmonary artery catheter is placed and the following results are obtained: PAP 42/28, CVP 30, PCWP 24, CO 1.9, CI 1.1, SVR 2442. An intra-aortic balloon pump is placed, and the norepinephrine is immediately discontinued. Nitroprusside is started and the dose is gradually increased as tolerated. Within several hours, the patient's urine output improves and her cardiac index increases to 1.6. Although placement of a LV assist device is considered, her hemodynamics continue to improve overnight with the afterload reduction provided by nitroprusside and aggressive diuresis.

The intra-aortic balloon pump is discontinued 2 days later and her respiratory support is able to be decreased. The patient is transitioned from nitroprusside to captopril, hydralazine and isosorbide dinitrate for afterload reduction and is successfully extubated 2 days later. Upon further improvement, low-dose carvedilol is added.

At the time of discharge her LV ejection fraction remains 10% but her right-ventricular (RV) function has significantly improved. She is ambulatory, fully alert and oriented, and denies dyspnea with mild exertion. She is euvolemic on exam with normalization of all lab values. She is discharged on a medical regimen of carvedilol, captopril, spironolactone, and oral furosemide with scheduled follow up in heart failure clinic.

CCU TIPS

- Postpartum cardiomyopthy frequently presents as fulminant failure and may require prolonged intensive-care-unit admission with supportive therapy.
- Early placement of a pulmonary artery catheter in the setting of fulminant heart failure can rapidly facilitate appropriate vasoactive therapies.

EXPERT COMMENTARY

Postpartum cardiomyopathy can present in a life-threatening fashion, with prompt diagnosis and full-court press therapy essential. Fortunately, in a majority of cases, if management is initiated promptly there is ultimately full recovery of myocardial function.

INDEX

NOTE: Page numbers followed by f indicate figures; t indicates tables.

Atropine
  in bradyarrhythmias, 153, 156
  post-coronary intervention, 51
Autograft valves, 105

B

Benzodiazepines, use in the CCU,
  282, 283*t*
Beta-blockers
  acute aortic insufficiency, 71
  constrictive pericarditis, 179
  mitral stenosis, 74
  NSTEMI, 28, 32–33
  STEMI, 23
  wide-complex tachycardia, 134
Bileaflet-tilting-disk valve, 105, 107*f*
Bilevel-positive airway pressure, 272
Bivalirudin
  NSTEMI, 33
  post-coronary intervention, 51
Blood transfusion, post-coronary
  intervention, 51
Bone marrow transplant, giant cell
  myocarditis and, 309–313,
  310–313*f*
Bosentan, pulmonary hypertension,
  209
Bradyarrhythmias, 152–159
  acute management, 153
  aortic dissection and, 169
  clinical presentation tips, 158
  complications, 158
  diagnostic tests, 156–157*f*
  differential diagnosis, 154
  discharge, 158
  medical management, 156–157
  physical exam, 152
  risk factors, 155
Bradycardia, hemodynamically
  significant, indication for
  temporary transvenous
  pacing, 244

Brockenbrough's sign, 215, 217*f*
Brugada criteria, 147, 148*f*
Brugada syndrome, 135, 138*f*

C

Caged-ball valves, 105, 107*f*
Calcium-channel blocker (CCB),
  pulmonary hypertension, 209
CardiacAssist Tandem Heart,
  225–226
Cardiac biomarkers, diagnosis
  NSTEMI, 31, 31*t*
  right-ventricular failure, 197
  STEMI, 22
Cardiac catheterization
  hypertrophic cardiomyopathy, 215,
  216–217*f*
  mitral regurgitation, 82
  STEMI, 22
Cardiac tamponade
  pericardiocentesis, 248
  in post-coronary intervention, 56
Cardiogenic shock, mitral stenosis
  and, 78
Cardiomyopathy. *see also* Heart failure
  (HF)
  hypertrophic, 212–219
  hypertrophic obstructive, 137–138
  ischemic and nonischemic,
  187–193
  postpartum, case report, 320–321
Cardiopulmonary resuscitation
  (CPR), wide-complex
  tachycardia, 133, 147
Cardioversion, 252–255
  atrial fibrillation in mitral
  stenosis, 75
  basic principles/definitions,
  253–254
  complications, 255
  contraindications, 252
  hypertrophic cardiomyopathy, 213

use in acute myocardial infarction, 39, 42
Left-ventricular assist device, MCS and transplant, 220–229
Left-ventricular free-wall rupture, 37
  acute management, 38–39
  clinical presentation, 30
  diagnostic tests, 40
  medical management, 41–42
  physical examination, 39–40
  surgical management, 42
Left-ventricular pump failure, 37
  acute management, 38–39
  clinical presentation, 39
  diagnostic tests, 40
  medical management, 41–42
  physical examination, 39
  surgical management, 41–42
Left-ventricular thrombus, LVAD for MCS and transplant, 226
Lepirudin, post-coronary intervention, 51
Lidocaine, wide-complex tachycardia, 133
Limb ischemia, IABP treatment and, 269
Long-QT syndrome, 135
Lorazepam, use in the CCU, 282, 283t
Low-molecular-weight heparin, for NSTEMI, 33

M

Macrolides, cause of WCT, 136t
Magnetic resonance imaging (MRI)
  constrictive pericarditis, 179, 182
  heart failure, 191
  hypertrophic cardiomyopathy, 215
  infective endocarditis, 98, 100
  pulmonary hypertension, 203, 208
  right-ventricular failure, 195
Malabsorption, nutrition in the CCU, 292

Malperfusion syndrome, aortic dissection and, 169
MAZE procedure, atrial fibrillation with mitral regurgitation, 86
McConnell's sign, 197
Mechanical circulatory support (MCS)
  acute management, 221–222
  complications, 226
  diagnostic tests, 220–223
  discharge, 227
  heart transplantation and, 220–229
  technologies used for, 223–226
Mechanical ventilation, 271–280
  acute management, 273
  complications, 272
  effects on cardiovascular system, 271–272
  inability to wean, 276
  initiation, 274f
  noninvasive, 272
  paralytic agents, 277, 279f
  sedation with, 277, 278f
  troubleshooting, 275
  weaning from, 275–276
Metoprolol
  acute aortic syndromes, 164
  hypertrophic cardiomyopathy, 213
  narrow complex tachycardia, 122
  for STEMI, 16
Midazolam, use in the CCU, 282, 283t
Milrinone, use in heart failure, 188, 191
Mitral regurgitation (MR), 36–37, 81–90
  acute management, 38–39, 82–83
  clinical presentation, 39, 81, 88
  complications, 88
  diagnostic tests, 40, 84–85
  differential diagnosis, 84
  discharge, 89
  etiologies, 85
  medical management, 41–42, 86–87